Christian and Faith-based Counseling for Brain Injury

Christian and Faith-based Counseling for Brain Injury: Techniques for Survivors and Families reflects Dr. Deana Adams' long-time academic research, teaching, and professional practice in working with brain injury survivors and their families. Her book is timely, relevant, and fills a gap specifically in Christian and faith-based compassionate counseling for persons surviving brain injury and their families.

– Rev. Dr. Helen T. Boursier, Ph.D.,
Author, Educator, Advocate, Ordained Minister

Christian and Faith-based Counseling for Brain Injury is the first book of its kind to offer faith-based therapy to address the emotional, cognitive, and mental health needs of individuals who have suffered a traumatic brain injury (TBI). A highly researched piece of work, the book puts forth an innovative and effective method not only for addressing the challenges of a life-changing injury but also for creating a sense of purpose.

Through the nuances of faith-based counseling, this book focuses on the spiritual and existential aspects of understanding the diagnosis and creating a purpose post-injury. It examines how brain injury can affect an individual by exploring the deficits of brain injury, the impact of brain injury, and the challenges specific to damage to certain brain lobes. It also describes the mental health issues, such as depression, anxiety, grief, anger, and posttraumatic stress, that can affect both the survivor and their family members. Offering targeted counseling techniques and adaptive strategies, it shows how faith-based counselors can effectively treat brain injury.

This book is valuable reading for all individuals invested in providing support to the TBI community. It is aimed at counselors, lay counselors, healthcare professionals, social workers, psychotherapists, seminary students, and upper-level graduate students. It will further be of use to clinicians working in the outpatient level of care and private practice settings.

Deana Adams, PhD, LPC-S, is the executive director of Hope Behavioral Health, a private practice specializing in traumatic brain injury. As the president and founder of Hope After Brain Injury, Dr. Adams speaks nationally and internationally, sharing insights on how to effectively counsel and facilitate successful recovery for those affected by brain injury.

Christian and Faith-based Counseling for Brain Injury

Techniques for Survivors and Families

Deana Adams

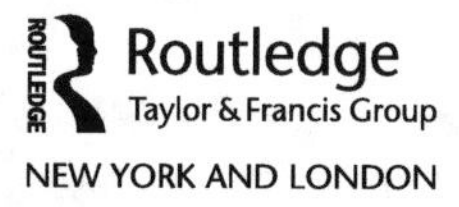

NEW YORK AND LONDON

Cover image: © Getty Images
First published 2023
by Routledge
605 Third Avenue, New York, NY 10158

and by Routledge
4 Park Square, Milton Park, Abingdon, Oxon, OX14 4RN

Routledge is an imprint of the Taylor & Francis Group, an informa business

© 2023 Deana Adams

The right of Deana Adams to be identified as author of this work has been asserted in accordance with sections 77 and 78 of the Copyright, Designs and Patents Act 1988.

All rights reserved. No part of this book may be reprinted or reproduced or utilised in any form or by any electronic, mechanical, or other means, now known or hereafter invented, including photocopying and recording, or in any information storage or retrieval system, without permission in writing from the publishers.

Trademark notice: Product or corporate names may be trademarks or registered trademarks, and are used only for identification and explanation without intent to infringe.

ISBN: 9781032295107 (hbk)
ISBN: 9781032292656 (pbk)
ISBN: 9781003301912 (ebk)

DOI: 10.4324/9781003301912

Typeset in Bembo
by Apex CoVantage, LLC

Contents

Figures

Foreword

The earliest written evidence of brain injuries is documented in Egypt in the Edwin Smith Papyrus, 3,000–2,500 BC, when the pyramids were built – the first medical document recognized in the history of medicine.

But it is only in recent years that traumatic brain injury (TBI) has been given a name and notoriety.

Due to high numbers of traumatic brain injury among active and retired professional football players in the United States, the National Football League established a concussion protocol in 2009, which has since been updated several times. Most sports have embraced similar safeguards. Regularly in the news today, we hear of athletes being sidelined for their protection because of all that is being learned about the life-altering consequences of TBI.

My personal connection to someone facing a "new normal" after excessive brain damage was an interview in 2008 for *100 Huntley Street*, a daily Canadian Christian television program. My guest, Patti Foster, nearly died in 2002 after a devastating car crash in Texas that left her in a coma for six weeks. She lives as a trophy of God's grace, helping and encouraging other victims of TBI and their friends and families. God's Spirit was at work when Dr. Deana Adams reconnected with the woman, who was not expected to walk or talk again. Deana had been working with trauma since 1991 and had seen its impact on lives as a first responder beginning in 1995. She began brain injury counseling in 2008 but became inspired to specialize in working with brain injury survivors. Launching Hope After Brain Injury in 2013, Deana has traveled around the globe, often speaking along with Patti to healthcare providers, survivors, and caregivers. These groups are all involved in working through the struggles and finding the path to hope, as you will read in the diverse case studies that follow.

In 2017, Deana and Patti came to Canada for a conference on TBI. It was a joy to have them stay in my home, and they complemented each other so well on our national Christian TV broadcast. But the Author of Life had an agenda that left us in awe. We were able to meet with two young women who were living with dramatic limitations, both as a result of serious brain injury in a car accident. These unplanned ministries to survivors and their family members were gifts from God, who engaged the expertise of the dynamic duo and poured His compassion through them.

This book is the first of its kind, and it could not be more timely. I have people eagerly waiting for their copy of *Christian and Faith-Based Counseling for Brain Injury: Techniques for Survivors and Families*.

> Now may God, the inspiration and fountain of hope, fill you to overflowing with uncontainable joy and perfect peace as you trust in him. And may the power of the Holy Spirit continually surround your life with his superabundance until you radiate with hope!
>
> Romans 15:13 (The Passion Translation, TPT)

Moira Brown
Broadcaster, Author, Speaker
Burlington, Ontario
Canada

Preface

Being starstruck has never been an issue for me until brain injury came into my life. Each time I meet a survivor of brain injury, a caregiver, or a healthcare professional specializing in brain injury, my stomach jumps into my chest. They are heroes to me. And, in my opinion, they are this world's best resource for resilience. In this book, I share case studies of clients with whom I have worked. Their names have been changed to protect their anonymity. I trust that their stories will resonate with the reader, offering hope and encouragement from a counselor blessed to work with this special population.

As I have gotten older, I have grown to appreciate the legacy of my family members. I come from a long line of medicine and ministry. My mom's side of the family were all in the medical field. My dad's side of the family were all ministers. So it came naturally for me to consider counseling as a vocation. My three homes were our house, the church, and the hospital. At age 7, I accepted Christ into my heart and became a Christian. When I was 21 years old, I dedicated my life to full-time Christian service as a Christian counselor. Working with individuals who struggle with mental health issues was my purpose and passion. In 1995, I was invited to be a first responder to the Oklahoma City (OKC) bombing, where I spent several days working with a local church and a hospital whose parishioners and staff suffered unbelievable trauma from the bombing and ongoing crime scene. Upon my return home, I was asked to volunteer as a police chaplain, which I did with three cities in the Dallas/Fort Worth area. I became a first responder to high-profile crime scenes and disasters.

Everything changed in 2008. While at a friend's house in East Texas, I re-met Patti Foster. I say re-met because she and I had originally met after the OKC bombing when she interviewed me on her radio program. She was a Christian radio host in Tyler, Texas. In 2002, Patti was in a horrific traffic accident and suffered a traumatic brain injury (TBI). At that meeting in 2008, she shared with me and her extended family, what it was like to live with a TBI. Up until that point, I was not aware of brain injury or its ramifications. In fact, at that time not many laypeople even knew what a TBI was. As we talked, I heard God speak to my heart that working with TBI was what I was going to do for the rest of my life. In 2013, Hope After Brain Injury (HABI) was established as the first faith-based, non-profit organization for brain injury. Since that time, I have served as the president and founder of HABI and have worked diligently in private practice with the brain injury community. Working as a licensed professional counselor-supervisor and Christian counselor, I have found that there are limited resources for treating brain injury in an outpatient setting. This book is meant to start a conversation on how to effectively counsel this community from a Christian and faith-based perspective. It is not meant to be the final word. My prayer is for God to show you his truth, understanding, and wisdom in counseling the brain injury population that they may be encouraged, equipped, and educated to reach their optimum potential and purpose.

Deana Adams

Acknowledgments

Success is incumbent on the shoulders on whom we stand. From my family, to the counseling world, to the brain injury world, I have been honored to work with giants in the field. My first hero, I never met. My paternal grandfather, Ernest Hancock, was an itinerant pastor who authored several books, led churches, hosted a radio program, and shared the Gospel throughout North Carolina. Although he passed away before I was born, I feel his influence today. I am very appreciative of my family who have encouraged me along the way. My husband, Rick, has been my stay and loving companion through the years. My father and mother, Philip and Wanda Hancock, have never wavered in their love, support, and belief in my work. Thanks to my friends and family who have encouraged me along the way and have been my virtual and in-person cheerleaders! I would like to extend my great appreciation to Patti Foster for sharing her inspiring story of recovery from a severe traumatic brain injury and her life today. I wish to offer my great appreciation to Judy Foster, Patti's mother, who shared her experiences as the mother of a victim of a severe traumatic brain injury.

I have had the honor of meeting and working with several professionals. Jennie Ponsford of Melbourne, Australia, encouraged me to write at the beginning of my career. Joseph Fins, Jeffrey Kreutzer, Kathleen Bell, Randi Dubiel, Mary Carlile, Marie Dahdah, Simon Driver, Surendra Barshikar, Andrew Maas, Karen Brewer-Mixon, Wynona Elder, Helen T. Boursier, Larry Ashlock, Karen Bullock, Mike and Mary Stedham, Moira Brown, and Norman Wright have all contributed as mentors, encouragers, and inspirations in my work as a counselor with brain injury survivors and their families. I am forever grateful to each of you.

I owe huge gratitude to Lucy Kennedy and Lakshay Gaba from Routledge Press for their kindness and professional guidance in writing this book. Their gentle and steadfast editorial expertise has been amazing.

Finally, I will forever be in debt to each of the survivors and family members who have shared their lives with me and trusted me to help them along their journey. You have my heart.

Deana Adams

1 Christian and Faith-Based Counseling Defined

Christian Counseling

Although a relatively new therapy model for brain injury, Christian counseling shows promise in its practice with survivors of traumatic brain injury (TBI) and their family members who recognize the spiritual aspect of recovery. The following is a brief history of the formation of Christian counseling. Both the Old Testament and New Testament of the Bible offer material of psychological import. Johnson and Jones (2000) state that, within the Christian tradition, the "Bible's reflections on human nature have always been accorded a unique authority." After the New Testament era, the psychological contributions of philosophers such as Aristotle and Plato influenced the theorizing of Christians for the next 1,400 years. However, according to Johnson and Jones (2000), Augustine provided the "best example in the early church of psychological reflection." Strongly influenced by Augustine, Thomas Aquinas captured the Augustinian and Aristotelian traditions and created a body of psychological thought covering emotions, intellect, will, vices, and virtues. After the Middle Ages, Søren Kierkegaard, who considered himself a Christian psychologist, "contributed some of the most profound theoretical psychological works ever written from a Christian or non-Christian standpoint" (Johnson & Jones, 2000). Thus, he could be considered the "father" of the modern approach to psychological theory and therapy. In 1903, William James, the father of American psychology, delved into the psychology of religion.

Wilhelm Wundt, a German philosopher and psychologist from the nineteenth century, is considered the father of experimental psychology. Wundt believed that psychology should be concerned with conscious awareness. His experiments were met with enthusiasm, especially in the United States by E.B. Titchener. His structuralism and introspection focused on breaking down mental processes into their most basic components of consciousness. Austrian psychiatrist Sigmund Freud claimed that it was not even possible for an individual to accurately observe his own mental life. Functionalism, founded by William James and studied by John Dewey, James Angell, and Harvey Carr, "helped shift the emphasis in psychology away from inner consciousness and toward the investigation of overt actions" (Collins, 1977). The introduction of behaviorism by John B. Watson moved psychology from introspection to an objective,

DOI: 10.4324/9781003301912-1

experimental branch of science. Behaviorism assumes that everything can be measured or quantified and that all scientific observations are objective. The American actress Mariette Hartley was John Watson's maternal granddaughter. In her book *Breaking the Silence* (2010), she described the adverse effects of behaviorism on her upbringing. She stated that her grandfather believed that "children were to be taken from mothers during their third or fourth week; if not, attachments were bound to develop." She continued, "children should never be kissed, hugged, or allowed to sit on their laps. If there should be kissing, let it be on the forehead." Parents were to be perfectly objective and kindly. Sadly, Hartley's mother and her siblings grew up "under a microscope, innocent receptacles of Grandfather's theories, conjectures, and absolutes." Of Watson's five children, three attempted suicide (one succeeded), and Mariette struggled with psychological issues. Most of the behaviorists studied human behavior as it responds to a stimulus. Unfortunately, by the late 1920s, psychology did not have an accepted behavioral principle. The positive influence of behaviorism is that it developed several objective and reliable experimental methods. B.F. Skinner regarded himself as a radical behaviorist and believed in observing behavior and describing how the observable stimuli created observable responses.

Freud's psychoanalysis theory contradicted the strict behaviorist tenet. He believed that all behavior is caused by unconscious mental processes. Psychoanalysis sought to uncover the unconscious causes. In his paper "A Religious Experience," Freud shared a letter from an American physician who "had heard a voice" that spoke to him, which led to a personal experience with God and Jesus Christ. He hoped that Freud would have an open mind to see God reveal the truth to his soul. Freud responded by politely saying,

> God had not done so much for me. He had never allowed me to hear an inner voice; and if, in view of my age, he did not make haste, it would not be my fault if I remained to the end of my life what I now was – "an infidel Jew."
>
> (Capps, 2001)

Alfred Adler, the father of individual psychology, expanded Freud's theory, stressing the importance of social interaction in behavior. Carl Jung, founder of analytic psychology, believed that people wear masks or personas to protect themselves in public. He extended his theory to consider folklore, myth, and religious symbolism (Collins, 1977). He espoused that the collective unconscious, the study of archetypes over space and time, was common to all humankind.

The second half of the twentieth century ushered *modern* psychology that separated psychology from theology and philosophy. It was not until after World War II "that conservative Protestants began to move out of their cultural ghettos and think more seriously about how their faith bears on the sciences and arts" (Johnson & Jones, 2000). In 1960, Clyde Narramore published an influential book, *The Psychology of Counseling: Professional Techniques for Pastors, Teachers, Youth Leaders and All Who Are Engaged in the Incomparable Art of Counseling*, outlining the Christian approach to counseling that blended scripture with Carl Rogers' person-centered therapy. In 1970, Jay Adams, author of *Competent to Counsel*, urged Christian counselors to practice "nouthetic counseling," which was to focus solely on the Bible and sin. Adams saw the Bible's way of counseling "as radically dependent on the work of the Holy Spirit to apply the Word of God to people's lives: the promises encourage and empower, the commands convict and guide, and the stories make application" (Powlison, 2005). Biblically based (formerly nouthetic) counseling focuses on the client coming to know Jesus Christ as his/her Lord and Savior first and foremost. Adams believed that pastors should be the primary counselors in the Christian community. In 2005, John MacArthur wrote *Counseling: How to Counsel Biblically*, in which he presents "a system of biblical truth that brings together people, their problems, and the living God." He states that the Bible is the counseling authority, the church should provide counseling as a basic ministry, and God's people should be trained to counsel effectively (MacArthur, 2005). Biblical counseling according to MacArthur should be biblical, practical, and easily understood. A skilled counselor is one "who carefully, prayerfully, and faithfully applies the divine spiritual resources to the process of sanctification, shaping another into the image of Jesus Christ" (MacArthur, 2005). MacArthur did not agree with Christian psychology, believing that it "is an attempt to harmonize two inherently contradictory systems of thought. Modern psychology and the Bible cannot be blended without serious compromise to or utter abandonment of the principle of Scripture's sufficiency."

In the latter 1970s, several psychologists attempted to study the overlap between theology and psychology. John Carter, Bruce Narramore (nephew of Clyde Narramore), Larry Crabb, and Gary Collins suggested an alternative integration approach. In his book *The Rebuilding of Psychology: An Integration of Psychology and Christianity*, Collins (1977) stated that the integration model of Christian counseling is consistent with the Bible and the general application of psychological sciences and professions. The goal of the Christian counselor is "to combine the special revelation of God's word with the general revelation studied by the psychological sciences and professions" (Narramore, 1973). Collins stated that, historically, psychology did not show much interest in religion; "science has tried to abandon religion and traditional theological tenets, it has not been able to eliminate beliefs, values, and philosophical assumptions" (Collins, 1977). The integration approach "tends to be more willing to criticize psychology in its modern form and to ask whether its findings are genuinely compatible with Scripture" (Johnson & Jones, 2000).

By the 1980s, evangelical clinicians such as James Dobson, Frank Minirth, and Paul Meier were hosting Christian radio programs addressing psychological issues, especially recovery from alcohol and substance abuse, from a Christian perspective. In 1985, Robert McGee authored *The Search for Significance*, which focused on how thoughts affect one's emotional, relational, and spiritual development. The book was the basis and curriculum for RAPHA Christ-Centered Hospital and Counseling Care. Minirth-Meier and New Life Treatment centers also created inpatient mental health and substance abuse treatment programs.

A group of Christian counselors, currently headed by Dr. Tim Clinton, started the American Association of Christian Counselors, which focuses solely on counseling from a conservative theological approach. To date, it is considered the largest, faith-based, mental health organization, offering a robust collection of counseling resources aimed at serving Christian counselors, pastors, and lay counselors.

The integration model is the foundation on which I base my Christian counseling approach in working with survivors of brain injury and their family members. Assumptions that form the basis for the Christian counseling approach to working with survivors of TBI and their families are as follows:

1 God exists and is the source of all truth.
2 We are made in the image of God and therefore are of inherent worth.
3 Every life, no matter the degree of impairment or health, embodies hope and purpose.
4 Science and scripture are complementary.
5 Christian counseling follows the tenets of scripture.

God Exists and Is the Source of All Truth

Truth, according to most theologians, is assumed through general revelation and special revelation of God. General or natural revelation refers to the truth God reveals through nature, science, history, observation, logical deduction, or empirical evidence. Due to the limits of such knowledge through inadequate methodologies, biased perceptions, or poor comprehension, general revelation is considered to be incomplete (Collins, 1977). Special revelation refers to the authority of the Bible. Christians believe that scripture is the God-inspired message that is trustworthy and complete (2 Timothy 3:16 English Standard Version, ESV). Collins (1977) explains that special revelation should accept "the facts of history and conclusions of established science, [have] the greatest internal consistency, [give] the most complete explanation of the 'unknown' and otherwise unknowable things about life and [have] the fewest translation inaccuracies or obvious errors." The Trinity of God the Father, God the Son, and God the Spirit are truth in the scripture (see John 14:6 New International Version (NIV), John 16:13 NIV, Psalm 119:160 NIV, John 1:14 ESV, John 14:17 NIV, and John 15:26 NIV). We access this truth by reading the Bible, praying, and meditating on His word.

We Are Made in the Image of God and Therefore Are of Inherent Worth

The *imago Dei*, the image of God, substantiates the significance and importance of every human being. The NIV of Genesis 1:27 says, "So God created mankind in his own image, in the image of God he created them; male and female he created them." Christian ethicist T.B. Maston (1967) wrote that the *imago Dei* was "the basis for the dignity and worth of man, a dignity that belongs to all men." The effects of brain injury do not negate or eliminate the significance, importance, value, or dignity belonging to each survivor and family member.

Every Life, No Matter the Degree of Impairment or Health, Embodies Hope and Purpose

Jeremiah 29:11 (English Standard Version, ESV) states, "For I know the plans I have for you, declares the Lord, plans for welfare and not for evil, to give you a future and a hope." Job 42:2 (ESV) says, "I know that you can do all things, and that no purpose of yours can be thwarted." Ephesians 2:10 (ESV) states that "we are his workmanship, created in Christ Jesus for good works, which God prepared beforehand, that we should walk in them." These are but a few verses in the Bible that proclaim that everyone has purpose. While brain injury affects the body and its physiology, it does not affect the spirit. There is no caveat or exception to this truth. In other words, whether a person is healthy or suffering from a chronic illness or brain injury, s/he still has purpose. In a recent conversation I had with Dr. Andrew Maas (personal communication, March 3, 2016), a neurosurgeon from Belgium, he stated that hope after a brain injury "is as essential as breath." Additionally, brain injury recovery is not only possible but also lifelong. With the research verifying the process of neuroplasticity, it is now believed that the brain continues to create new pathways in place of neurons damaged in brain injury.

Science and Scripture Are Complementary

The Bible is sufficient for spiritual wholeness. However, an omniscient God may instill His truth in scientific, rehabilitative, and other research whereby we may glean understanding and practice. Philosopher Arthur Holmes (1971) stated that there are three ways in which the fields of religion and science interrelate. First, both religion and science use models to explain reality. To know about humans, one uses a variety of models such as chemistry, sociology, physiology, and the humanities. To know about Christ, one studies parables, analogies, and word pictures from the Bible (Collins, 1977). Holmes' second point was that any conflict between the two was not ultimately over empirical facts but between the assumptions upon which the facts were built. His final thought concluded that science and every other human endeavor find their ultimate meaning in religion. Mathematician and physicist Lord William Tomson Kelvin stated in a lecture at the University College Association of London in 1903, "Let nobody be afraid of true freedom of thought. Let us be free in thought and criticism, but with freedom we are bound to come to the conclusion that science is not antagonistic but is a help to religion" (Holmes, 1916).

Christian Counseling Follows the Tenets of Scripture

Integrative Christian counseling allows the clinician to make use of therapeutic tools and established skills with the awareness of God's character, presence, and direction within the therapeutic relationship. Gordon Allport (1950), one of the most influential psychologists in the twentieth century, stated that "love is incomparably the greatest psychotherapeutic agent. . . . The Christian religion offers an interpretation of life and a rule of life based wholly upon love. It calls attention again and again to this fundamental groundwork." While biblical counseling focuses primarily on an individual's conversion, integrative Christian counseling acknowledges God's existence and relevance to the therapeutic process. It also recognizes the current research in a variety of fields that contribute to health and healing. Collins (1977) explained further that "people are biological organisms whose behavior and emotions largely depend on their individual physiology and environmental influences." People are also influenced "by supernatural forces, freed from sin's penalty by acceptance of Jesus Christ, are protected by a loving God, and are guided by his Holy Spirit" (Collins, 1977).

Christian Counseling Praxis

The Apostle Paul opened his second letter to the Corinthians with thanksgiving to God, the Father of Jesus Christ, for delivering him from tribulation and giving him the ability to comfort others as he was comforted by God. 2 Corinthians 1:3–4 NIV says "Praise be to the God and Father of the Lord Jesus Christ, the Father of compassion and the God of all comfort, who comforts us in all our troubles, so that we can comfort those in any trouble with the comfort we ourselves receive from God." The Greek word for comfort in this passage was *parakalĕō*, meaning to be of good comfort, exhort, entreat, and pray. The Greek word used for affliction was *thlipsis*, meaning anguish, afflicted, burdened, and persecution. Survivors of brain injury and their family members and caregivers understand the intricacies of affliction. Christians are called to walk with the afflicted. Part of the Compline prayer says "pity the afflicted," meaning to have compassion and share in someone's sadness or suffering. Anglican priest Tish Warren stated in her book, *Prayer in the Night*, that "we ask that God might feel what we feel, to enter into the dark room in which we find ourselves and sit with us in our pain and vulnerability." Survivors experience a wide variety of comforters, such as nurses, neuropsychologists, physical therapists, speech therapists, occupational therapists, physical medicine and rehabilitation physicians, vocational counselors, and nutritionists, to name a few. The passage in 2 Corinthians encapsulates the reality that one who suffers and who is afflicted can comfort others in a special way that s/he knows through his/her own suffering. It is assumptive that the God of all comfort equips survivors of TBI and their family members with how to comfort one another as they cope daily with the effects of TBI.

Truax and Carkhuff (2007) stated that an effective counselor should exhibit three qualities: empathic understanding, nonpossessive warmth, and genuineness or authenticity. Simply, the role of a Christian counselor is to comfort, educate, equip, and encourage with the truths of God. The underpinning of an effective counselor is sharing one's knowledge and support fueled by the love of God. Romans 5:5 (New Century Version, NCV) says, "And this hope will never disappoint us, because God has poured out his love to fill our hearts. He gave us his love through the Holy Spirit, whom God has given us." A Christian counseling praxis begins with the understanding that God is an integral part of the healing process. One needs to prepare spiritually, physically, psychologically, and mentally to be an effective Christian counselor, especially for the brain injury population. Spiritual preparation is inviting the Holy Spirit into the counseling room before and throughout every session. Praying for wisdom, hope, and timely words welcomes the truth of God to be expressed in a kind and respectful manner. Physical preparation ensures the counselor has given him/herself the needed nutrition, exercise, and rest to fully function in his/her role each day. Additionally, it is important to create a healthy schedule whereby one creates space or breaks within the schedule of each day. Psychological or emotional preparation may include having a personal therapist or counselor whom one may employ as support. Practicing good boundaries and staying objective help the counselor to insulate him/herself against burnout or compassion fatigue. Mental preparation, namely, educating oneself about brain injury and its effects, trajectories, treatments, best practices, and prognoses is foundational to one's effectiveness as a counselor for the brain injury population. To create coping strategies, instill hope for healing and recovery, and journey with the survivors through the process of grieving the loss of their pre-injury functioning and to encourage them toward post-injury quality of life are the overall goals. Innate in this approach is the belief that God is intricately involved in the recovery process. Techniques include utilizing the latest research (and recognizing the limitations thereof), active listening, educating about brain injury, and assisting the survivor and family as they move through various stages of recovery. The stages of treatment and stages of grief, along with navigating the emotional upheavals of brain injury toward optimum recovery, are essential goals of counseling. Because people are made in the image of God, the *imago Dei*, He is inherently invested in their becoming the best they can be, despite and during affliction.

Spirituality, Religion, and No Faith

Religion and spirituality appear to play a significant role as a means of coping with brain injury and its accompanying stressors. Waldron-Perrine et al. (2011) stated that research has shown that there is a link between one's religious practices and rehabilitation outcomes. Spirituality and religion may occur within the same construct or separately, depending on one's belief system. In other words, people may experience spirituality within a religious context or experience spirituality without a religious context. Johnstone et al. (2016) utilized the Brief Multidimensional Measure of Religiousness/Spirituality (BMMRS) to determine the factor structure for diverse cultures, ethnicities, and religions. They included 109 survivors of TBI (at least 6 months post-injury) in their study. They defined the primary measures of religiousness as private religious experiences (religious activities), organizational religiousness (frequency of involvement in formal religious events), and religious support (the degree to which individuals feel supported, helped, and comforted by their local congregations). They identified primary measures of spirituality as daily spiritual practices, meaning, values/beliefs, and forgiveness. The results from their study found that survivors of TBI who felt closer to their higher power engaged more frequently in private religious experiences such as prayer, meditation, and ritual. This result may be due to the fact that individuals with TBI

> are relatively isolated due to increased functional disability and limited transportation and therefore may be unable to attend organized religious services. As a result, it may be that private religious practices are the primary method by which they can express their spiritual beliefs.
>
> (Johnstone et al., 2016)

An earlier study noted that, "for all faith traditions, the presence of positive and absence of negative personality traits are primary indicators of positive health (and primarily mental health)" (Johnston et al., 2012).

Religious or spiritual well-being (a meaningful relationship with God) and existential well-being (the general belief that one's life is meaningful or has purpose) were addressed in Waldron-Perrine et al.'s (2011) research. They found that, "[S]pecific facets of religious and spiritual belief systems play important and unique roles in predicting rehabilitation outcomes after TBI." They also stated that a sense of connectedness to a higher power "was more strongly predictive than were a nonreligious sense of meaning and purpose in life or engagement in religious activities." Their study documented that public religious practice was unrelated to rehabilitation outcome. Interestingly, however, "whereas religious well-being was beneficially related to all the rehabilitation outcomes, and uniquely so, existential well-being was not." They suggested that contentment with one's purpose and meaning in life may not project the person toward improvement. Additionally, "existential well-being was unrelated to general well-being and other health outcomes." They concluded, "given what is known about the paucity of social support resources after TBI, it is likely that religious support is an especially important resource in this population." Clinical implications include strong encouragement for those working with survivors of TBI to understand their worldview and incorporate those beliefs into rehabilitative care. Saunders et al. (2010) recommend that clinicians practice "spiritually conscious psychological care" that incorporates the client's belief system into his/her rehabilitative treatment.

Few studies have been done that address the role of atheism or no faith in rehabilitation. However, Wilkinson and Coleman (2009) studied a population of people over 60 in southern England who had religious beliefs and atheistic beliefs. In their study, they found that the participants were coping well with the aging process regardless of their beliefs. They stated that

> a strong atheistic belief system can fulfill the same role as a strong religious belief system in providing support, explanation, consultation and inspiration. It is postulated that the strength of people's beliefs and how those beliefs are used might have more influence on the efficacy of coping than the specific nature of the beliefs.

Recognizing the validity of this and other research, I will describe Christian, faith-based, and spiritual counseling techniques throughout this book to address the emotional, cognitive, and behavioral challenges of brain injury.

Conclusion

This chapter gave a history of Christian counseling and its variants such as biblical and nouthetic counseling. Also discussed were the specific assumptions that underpin the Christian counseling approach to brain injury. The praxis of Christian counseling was explained along with the need for proper spiritual, psychological, and physical preparation of the clinician. A Christian counselor is in part called "to care for the afflicted, to affirm the dignity of every human being as an image bearer of God" (Warren, 2021). Additional studies that supported religious, spiritual, atheistic, and existential beliefs as they pertain to coping skills for individuals with brain injury were addressed.

References

Allport, G. (1950). *The individual and his religion*. MacMillan Publishing.

Collins, G. (1977). *The rebuilding of psychology: An integration of psychology and Christianity*. Tyndale House Publishers.

Freud, S. (1928/2001). A religious experience. In D. Capps, (Ed.), *Freud and Freudians on religion* (pp. 58–61). Yale University.

Hartley, M. & Commire, A. (2010). *Breaking the silence*. Cavu Productions.

Holmes, A. (1916). The faith of the scientist. *The Biblical World, 48*, 3–7.

Holmes, A. (1971). *Faith seeks understanding: A Christian approach to knowledge*. Eerdmans.

Johnson, E., & Jones, S. (2000). A history of Christians in psychology. In E. Johnson & S. Jones (Eds.), *Psychology and Christianity: Four views* (pp. 11–53). InterVarsity Press.

Johnstone, B., Yoon, D., Cohen, D., Schoop, L., McCormack, G., Campbell, J., & Smith, M. (2012). Relationships among spirituality, religious practices, personality factors, and health for five different faith traditions. *Journal of Religion and Health, 51*, 1017–1041.

Johnstone, B., Bhushan, B., Hanks, R., Yoon, D., & Cohen, D. (2016). Factor structure of the Brief Multidimensional Measure of Religiousness/Spirituality in US and Indian samples with traumatic brain injury. *Journal of Religion and Health, 55*, 572–586.

MacArthur, J. (2005). *Counseling: How to counsel biblically*. Thomas Nelson.

Maston, T. (1967). *Biblical ethics: A guide to the ethical message of the scriptures from Genesis to Revelation*. Mercer University Press.

McGee, R. (1985). *The search for significance: We can build our self-worth on our ability to please others, or on the love and forgiveness of Jesus Christ*. Rapha Publishing.
Narramore, B. (1973). Perspectives on the integration of psychology and theology. *Journal of Psychology and Theology*, *1*, 3–17.
Powlison, D. (2005). Biblical counseling in recent times. In J. MacArthur (Ed.), *Counseling: How to counsel biblically* (pp. 18–30). Thomas Nelson.
Saunders, S., Miller, M., & Bright, M. (2010). Spiritually conscious psychological care. *Professional Psychology: Research and Practice*, *41*(5), 355–362. https://doi.org/10.1037/a0020953
Truax, C., & Carkhuff, R. (2007). *Toward effective counseling and psychotherapy: Training and practice*. Routledge.
Waldron-Perrine, B., Rapport, R., Hanks, R., Lumley, M., Meachen, S., & Hubbarth, P. (2011). Religion and spirituality in rehabilitation outcomes among individuals with traumatic brain injury. *Rehabilitation Psychology*, *56*(2), 107–116.
Warren, T. (2021). *Prayer in the night: For those who work or watch or weep*. InterVarsity Press.
Wilkinson, P., & Coleman, P. (2009). Strong beliefs and coping in old age: A case-based comparison of atheism and religious faith. *Ageing and Society*, *30*(2), 337–361. https://doi.org/10.1017/S0144686X09990353

2 Brain Injury Defined

Acquired Brain Injury Versus Traumatic Brain Injury

The term brain injury has been divided into two main categories: acquired brain injury (ABI) and traumatic brain injury (TBI). In some countries, acquired brain injury is the umbrella term under which traumatic brain injury sits. For example, Brain Injury Australia and Brain Injury British Columbia use ABI as the all-encompassing term for all brain injuries sustained after birth. The definition of TBI is often used synonymously with ABI; however, ABI is any injury to the brain after birth not associated with an external force. Most researchers identify TBI as a subset of ABI, along with brain tumors, strokes, cerebral hemorrhages, and brain aneurysms.

Traumatic brain injury is defined as "an alteration in brain function, or the evidence of brain pathology, caused by an external force" (Menon et al., 2010). Criteria for an alteration in brain function include the following:

- any period of loss of consciousness
- any loss of memory for events immediately before or after the injury
- neurologic deficits such as weakness, loss of balance, change in vision, paralysis, sensory loss, or aphasia
- any alteration in mental state at the time of the injury (confusion, disorientation, slowed thinking, etc.)

Evidence of brain pathology may include "visual, neuroradiologic [neuroimaging], laboratory confirmation of brain damage" (Menon et al., 2010). External force may include the head being struck by an object, the head striking an object, coup-contrecoup (back and forth motion when the brain hits one side of the skull and bounces to the opposite side of the skull), a foreign object penetrating the brain, forces from a blast or explosion, or other force yet to be defined.

The skull (cranium) encases the brain and comprises 22 bones, 21 of which are a single unit. The 22nd bone is the mandible (jaw), which is the only movable bone of the skull. The underside of the skull has sharp edges or ridges that can bump and bruise the surface of the brain. The brain itself weighs

DOI: 10.4324/9781003301912-2

approximately three pounds and is surrounded by the dura mater, arachnoid mater, and pia mater, which comprise the layer of thick, fibrous, connective tissue. Billions of nerve fibers run from one part of the brain to another. When the brain is injured, these fibers are stretched and damaged. The arteries and veins can leak blood, which causes the brain to swell. If there is a tear, blood can run out creating a bruise like one in any other part of the body.

Classification of Brain Injury

The classification of TBI was historically determined by the Glasgow Coma Scale (Teasdale & Jennett, 1974), a system used to assess coma and impaired consciousness. The physician assesses the eye-opening response (spontaneous blinking, response to verbal stimuli, response to pain, or no response), verbal response (oriented, confused conversation, inappropriate words, incomprehensible speech, or no speech), and motor response (obeys commands, purposeful movement to pain stimulus, withdrawal in response to pain, decorticate posturing where arms are flexed over the chest, decerebrate posturing, or no response) to determine the severity of the brain injury. Decerebrate posturing is an abnormal posture whereby the arms are extended to the sides of the body, the legs are straight, the toes are pointed downward, and the neck and head are arched backwards. Decorticate posturing is an abnormal posture whereby the body is stiff, the arms/wrists are bent towards the chest, the fists are clinched, and the legs are held out straight. Both types of posturing are indicative of severe damage to the brain. Severe brain injury is indicated by a score less than 8. Moderate brain injury is indicated by a score between 9 and 12, and mild brain injury is indicated by a score of 13–15.

More recently, three other classifications have come to be used as indicators of brain injury severity. These are posttraumatic amnesia (PTA), alteration of consciousness (AOC), and loss of consciousness (LOC). PTA is "a state of generalized cognitive disturbance characterized by confusion, disorientation, retrograde amnesia, inability to store new memories, and sometimes agitation and delusions" (Ponsford et al., 2014). PTA duration includes "the period of coma and is calculated from the moment of injury until the return of the capacity to store and retrieve new information" (Ponsford et al., 2014). If the individual has PTA for one day or less, it is considered a mild traumatic brain injury (mTBI). Moderate severity is marked by PTA of more than one and fewer than seven days. Severe traumatic brain injury is indicated by PTA longer than seven days. Alteration of consciousness "must be immediately related to trauma to the head" (Blyth & Bazarian, 2010). Symptoms of AOC may include looking or feeling dazed, confusion, the inability to think clearly or answer questions appropriately, and the inability to describe events before or after the injury. Mild traumatic injury is indicated by AOC from one minute up to 24 hours. Moderate and severe TBI are indicated with AOC of longer than 24 hours. Blyth and Bazarian (2010) stated that LOC requires "either loss of the function of both cerebral hemispheres or of the reticular activating system." The reticular activating system is a gatekeeper consisting of a bundle of nerves in the brainstem that filters out unnecessary information, thereby allowing in information needed by the conscious mind. Loss of consciousness of less than 30 minutes indicates a mTBI (Blyth & Bazarian, 2010). Moderate TBI is LOC greater than 30 minutes and fewer than 24 hours. Severe TBI is marked by LOC greater than 24 hours. Catastrophic brain injury is defined as "any brain injury that is expected to result in permanent loss of all brain function above the brain stem level" (Neal et al., 2018).

Classification and diagnosis of TBI are also dependent on neuroimaging. Due to recent advances in both structural and functional neuroimaging, it is now possible to better understand the type of TBI. Computed tomography (CT) is indicated for patients with a moderate or severe TBI (Le, Stiver, & Gean, 2012). CT is "useful in the detection of skull fractures, intracranial haematomas, large contusions, cerebral abscess, hygromas, brain swelling infarction, ventricular enlargement and atrophy" (Ponsford, 2013). Magnetic resonance imaging (MRI) is preferred over CT because of its superior sensitivity to older blood products and increased detection of damage to gray and white matter as well as lesions in the brainstem (Le, Stiver, & Gean, 2012). Other functional imaging techniques provide information regarding metabolic activity in various parts of the brain, although none are routinely available clinically (Ponsford 2013). These include positron emission tomography (PET), which measures regional metabolic rates of oxygen and glucose, single photon emission computer tomography (SPECT), which uses gamma-emitting isotopes to measure cerebral blood flow (Le, Stiver & Gean, 2012), and magnetic resonance spectroscopy (MRS), which measures metabolites as indicators of pathology (Ponsford, 2013).

Prevalence

Traumatic brain injury, once considered a "silent epidemic," affects approximately 69 million people and is now the greatest contributor to death and disability among all trauma-related injuries worldwide (Dewan et al., 2019). Traumatic brain injury is a major cause of death and disability in the United States, contributing to nearly 2.2% of all deaths (Taylor et al., 2017). More recently, in 2019 in the United States (US), 1.5–2 million people sustain a TBI each year [Centers for Disease Control and Prevention (CDC), 1999]. According to the TBI Surveillance Report of those affected by TBI, 223,135 were hospitalized and 64,362 died in 2020 (CDC, 2022). TBI continues to be the leading cause of death among young adults, children, and persons over the age of 75 (CDC, 2022). In 2014, there were approximately 2.87 million people admitted to the emergency room for TBI in the US (CDC, 2019). According to a CDC (2019) report, the prevalence of emergency department visits, hospitalizations, and deaths increased by 53% from 2006. Although in the US it is reported that women comprise approximately 40% of the general population experiencing emergency department visits, hospitalizations, or deaths related to TBI, they are reported to have a greater risk of TBI related to vehicle accidents, falls, and intimate partner violence (IPV), while experiencing worse post-injury outcomes than men (Munivenkatappa et al., 2016). These authors' research also reported that females had significantly higher rates of mild head injury and mortality. Biegon (2021) further describes that many of the victims of IPV experience severe attacks in the form of being hit, kicked, choked, beaten, burned, stabbed, or shot, and that many of the attacks are likely to result in TBI or anoxic brain injury due to abuser's targeting of the victim's face, head, and neck. Due to the numbers of women over 15 years old experiencing IPV, "there could be more than 31,000,000 women who have received a traumatic brain injury in the US today" (Biegon, 2021).

Dewan et al. (2019) researched the global impact of TBI across 66 countries. Their model indicated that between 64 and 74 million new cases of TBI will occur worldwide each year. According to Dewan et al. (2019), the US, Canada, and Europe reported the greatest incidence of TBI, while the African regions reported the lowest incidence. The greatest overall burden of TBI was reported in the Southeast Asian region and Western Pacific. The healthcare systems in low- to middle-income countries encounter three times as many total cases of TBI as those in high-income countries.

Prevalence is also divided by gender and age. Frost et al. (2013) found in their meta-analysis that approximately 12% of the general population of adults has a history of TBI with LOC. The odds of a "history of TBI resulting in the LOC are 2.2 times higher for males than females" (Frost et al., 2013). According to the TBI Surveillance report (2019), the highest number of TBI-related hospitalizations and deaths occurred in adults 75 years of age or older. Young children (0–4 years) and young adults (15–24 years) had among the highest number of emergency department visits (CDC, 2019). Interestingly, females have a higher incidence of concussions in sports than their male counterparts. Although the reason for the disparity is unclear, it is speculated that neck strength and gender-specific brain physiology contribute to these findings (Kegel & Lovell, 2011).

Types of Brain Injury

External Origin

Traumatic brain injury most often originates from an external force. Closed head injury, an open or penetrating head injury, diffuse axonal injury (DAI), crushing head injury, epidural hematoma, subdural hematoma, traumatic subarachnoid hemorrhage, and intraventricular hemorrhage are the most often identified. Closed head injury occurs when there is no break in the skin or skull nor an open wound. Normally, this happens when the head suddenly changes motion, whether due to acceleration (a car crash from behind) or deceleration (a car crash into a brick wall). As the head changes movement or rotates, the brain "is forced to follow the movements of the skull, and as it is a soft and jelly-like, it gets twisted in the process" (Gronwall et al., 2002). Coup-contrecoup

(French for "blow" and "counterblow") injury occurs when there is damage on two sides of the brain from one incident. Coup is the result of the direct impact, and contrecoup occurs when the brain hits the opposite side of the skull from the location of where the head is struck.

An open or penetrating brain injury occurs when the scalp and bone are penetrated, causing damage to the brain itself. Normally, acceleration is the cause, for example, being struck by a bullet or flying through a car window.

Diffuse axonal injury occurs when the brain shifts and rotates, causing a shearing or tearing of the long axons attached to the long nerves of the brain. Because of the nature of the injury, DAI is more widespread throughout the brain.

Crushing head injury is the least common type of TBI. The damage occurs when the brain and skull are crushed between two hard, stationary objects. For example, the head may be caught between the wheel of a car and the pavement or between a boat and the wharf.

Epidural hematoma is the result of an accumulation of blood between the skull and the outer layer of dura mater. Subdural hematoma occurs when there is a tear between the dura mater and the arachnoid layer. Traumatic subarachnoid hemorrhage is bleeding in the subarachnoid space of the brain between the arachnoid and pia mater. Intraventricular hemorrhage is bleeding inside and around the ventricles of the brain.

Carbon monoxide poisoning can produce different patterns of brain injury. Carbon monoxide is a toxic, colorless, and odorless gas that reduces the oxygen-carrying capacity of blood, causing tissue hypoxia (Lo et al., 2007). It replaces the oxygen in the bloodstream and causes the heart, brain, and body to become starved of oxygen. The results can be fatal. Symptoms of carbon monoxide poisoning are dizziness, fainting, nausea, chest pain, loss of muscle coordination, headache, shortness of breath, and mental confusion. In 2017, the worldwide cumulative incidence and mortality of carbon monoxide poisoning was estimated to cause 4.6 deaths per million, respectively (Mattiuzzi & Lippi, 2020).

Internal Origin

Strokes are divided into two categories: ischemic and hemorrhagic. Ischemic strokes are more common and occur due to a narrowing of the arterial openings and decreased blood flow to areas of the brain. Hemorrhagic strokes are less common and occur when a weakened blood vessel ruptures and bleeds into the surrounding brain tissue.

Other internal acquired brain injuries are caused by aneurysm, arteriovenous malformation, Chiari malformation, and cerebrospinal fluid (CSF) leakage. As blood passes through a weak spot in an artery or blood vessel, it causes the weakened area to balloon or bulge. The bulge is called an aneurysm, which can rupture and cause bleeding in the brain. An arteriovenous malformation is an abnormal cluster of blood vessels that also can rupture and cause bleeding in the brain. Chiari malformation occurs when the cerebellum bulges through the normal opening in the skull and joins the spinal canal, putting pressure on the brain and the spinal cord. Leakage can occur when cerebrospinal fluid escapes through a small hole or tear in the dura mater, causing the pressure in the brain and spinal cord to drop. This can cause headaches that are worse while sitting, light sensitivity, nausea, neck stiffness, and drainage from the ears or nose.

Causes of Brain Injury

The Centers for Disease Prevention and Control (1999) report that falls are the greatest cause of TBI in the elderly. The marked increase in the incidence of older adults has been called the "silver tsunami" (Corrigan et al., 2019). According to Taylor et al. (2017), in 2013 falls were the leading cause of TBI in the United States, accounting for 47.2% of all TBIs, followed by being struck by or against an object (15.4%) and motor vehicle crashes (13.7%). Motor vehicle accidents are the greatest cause of TBI-related hospitalizations, and violence (especially assaults that include firearms) is the leading cause of TBI-related deaths. Daughtery et al. (2019) reported that "suicide surpassed motor vehicle crashes as the leading category of TBI-related deaths during 2009–2011 and through 2015–2017."

Traumatic brain injury is considered the "signature injury" of the conflicts in Iraq and Afghanistan (Okie, 2005). Among post-9/11 veterans, rates of TBI have been estimated between 11% and 23% (Abraham et al., 2020). Agimi et al. (2020) found that of the 4,877 service members in their study, an estimated 65.6% were identified with severe TBI, 56.2% with penetrating TBI, 31.4% with moderate TBI, and 12.0% with mild TBI who were predicted to develop long-term disability. Blast injuries account for approximately 60% of military-related TBIs, of which 80% are considered mild TBIs (McKee & Robinson, 2014). Injury from explosive blasts "varies depending on the strength of the explosive; whether the injury occurs in an open field, or near buildings; or in a motor vehicle" (McKee & Robinson, 2014). Phillips (1986) subdivided blast injuries into three categories. Primary injury refers to the direct impact caused by the pressure changes of a blast. Secondary injury refers to the injury caused by objects put in motion by the blast. Tertiary injury refers to when a person is thrown by the blast, striking another object or the ground.

Traumatic brain injury is further divided into three categories. The primary injury occurs within two seconds whereby the brain is accelerated, decelerated, or rotated; nerve fibers are stretched, arteries and veins are torn, and it may occur with or without an open wound. The second injury occurs in the first hour when breathing is obstructed and the brain is deprived of oxygen. Also, blood loss lowers blood pressure and reduces the supply of blood and oxygen to the brain. The third injury occurs within 24–48 hours, whereby the brain swells and bruises, blood clots are formed, and posttraumatic hydrocephalus (circulation of fluid around the brain is blocked by scarring) develops (Gronwall et al., 2002).

Injury to the brain because of high acceleration and multiple or rotational impacts to the head in the context of sports contributes to approximately 15% of TBIs. Generally, the highest rates of TBI occur in hockey, rugby, equestrian activities, cycling, winter sports, and football (Theadom et al., 2014). In their study in New Zealand, Theadom et al. (2014) reported that up to 19% of TBIs were not recorded in medical notes. In the US, the incidence of sports-related TBI is estimated to range from 300,000 to 3.8 million cases per year (Winker et al., 2016). In Winkler et al.'s study, aquatic sports reported the fewest number of TBIs, while equestrian and related sports accounted for the greatest number of sports-related TBIs (45.2%). In people aged 18–29, roller sports such as roller skating and skateboarding contributed the most TBIs (33%). Of all the sports played in the United States, American football "is the sport associated with the greatest number of traumatic brain injuries, but it also has the largest number of participants" (Daneshvar et al., 2011).

Conclusion

Traumatic brain injury is a leading cause of death and disability in the United States, costing upward of $48 billion annually. Because of the potential severity of TBI, the multiple levels of care, and the economic cost, TBI is a significant public health burden in the US and internationally. This chapter gave an overview of acquired and traumatic brain injuries. The classification of TBI, its prevalence, the types of brain injury, and their causes were discussed. Special attention was given to gender differences and military-specific brain injuries. The next chapter will explore the stages of treatment, beginning with the initial injury through various levels of treatment to the transition from rehabilitation center to home. It begins with a case study of Patti Foster, a former radio personality who suffered a traumatic brain injury in a motor vehicle accident.

References

Abraham, T., Ono, S., Moriarty, H., Winter, L., Bender, R., Facundo, R., & True, G. (2020). Revealing the invisible emotion work of caregivers: A photovoice exploration of informal care provided by family caregivers for post-9/11 veterans with traumatic brain injuries. *Journal of Head Trauma Rehabilitation, 16*(1), 25–33.

Agimi, Y., Marion, D., Schwab, K., & Stout, K. (2020). Estimates of long-term disability among US service members with traumatic brain injury. *Journal of Head Trauma Rehabilitation, 36*(1), 1–9.

Biegon, A. (2021). Considering biological sex in traumatic brain injury. *Frontiers in Neurology, 12*, 1–12. https://doi.org/10.3389/fneur.2021.576366

Blyth, B., & Bazarian, J. (2010). Traumatic alterations in consciousness: Traumatic brain injury. *Emergency Medicine Clinics of North America, 28*(3), 571–594.

Centers for Disease Control and Prevention (2019). *Surveillance report of traumatic brain injury-related emergency department visits, hospitalizations, and deaths: United States 2014.* Centers for Disease Control and Prevention, U.S. Department of Health and Human Services.

Centers for Disease Control and Prevention (2022). *TBI surveillance report: United States 2018 and 2019*. Centers for Disease Control and Prevention, U.S. Department of Health and Human Services.

Corrigan, J., Harrison-Felix, C., & Haarbauer-Krupa, J. (2019). Epidemiology of traumatic brain injury. In J. Silver, T. McAllister, & D. Arciniegas (Eds.), *Textbook of traumatic brain injury* (3rd ed., pp. 3–24). American Psychiatric Association Publishing.

Daneshvar, D., Nowinski, C., McKee, A., & Cantu, R. (2011). The epidemiology of sport-related concussion. *Clinics in Sports Medicine, 30*(1), 1–17. https://doi.org/10.1016/j.csm.2010.08.006

Daughtery, J., Waltzman, D., Sarmiento, K., & Xu, L. (2019). Traumatic brain injury-related deaths by race/ethnicity, sex, intent, and mechanism of injury – United States, 2000–2017. *Morbidity and Mortality Weekly Report, 68*(46), 1050–1056.

Dewan, M., Rattani, A., Gupta, S., Baticulon, R., Ya-Ching, H., Punchak, M., Agrawal, A., Adelye, A., Shrime, M., Rubiano, A., Rosenfeld, J., & Park, K. (2019). Estimating the global incidence of traumatic brain injury. *Journal of Neurosurgery, 130*, 1080–1097.

Division of Acute Care, Rehabilitation Research, and Disability Prevention, National Center for Injury Prevention and Control, Centers for Disease Control and Prevention, U.S. Department of Health and Human Services (1999). *Traumatic brain injury in the United States: A report to Congress*. www.cdc.gov/traumaticbraininjury/pubs/tbi_report_to_congress.html

Frost, R., Farrer, T., Primosch, M., & Hedges, D. (2013). Prevalence of traumatic brain injury in the general adult population: A meta-analysis. *Neuroepidemiology, 40*, 154–159. https://doi.org/10.1159/000343275

Gronwall, D., Wrightson, P., & Waddell, P. (2002). *Head injury: The facts* (2nd ed.). Oxford University Press.

Kegel, N., & Lovell, M. (2011). Sports-related concussion: Identification and return-to-play decision-making. In F. Zollman (Ed.), *Manual of Traumatic Brain Injury Management* (pp. 58–64). Demos Medical Publishing.

Le, T., Stiver, S., & Gean, A. (2012). Imaging diagnosis of TBI. In J. Tsao (Ed.), *Traumatic brain injury: A clinician's guide to diagnosis, management, and rehabilitation* (pp. 15–48). Springer Science+Business Media. https://doi.org/10.1007/978-0-387-87887-4_2

Lo, C. P., Chen, S.Y., Lee, K.W., Chen, W. L., Chen, C.Y., Hsueh, C. J., & Huang, G. S. (2007). Brain injury after acute carbon monoxide poisoning: Early and late complications. *American Journal of Roentgenology, 189*(4), W205–W211. http://doi.org/10.2214/AJR.07.2425

Mattiuzzi, C., & Lippi, G. (2020). Worldwide epidemiology of carbon monoxide poisoning. *Human and Experimental Toxicology, 39*(4), 387–392. http://doi.org/10.1177/0960327119891214

McKee, A., & Robinson, M. (2014). *Military-related traumatic brain injury and neurodegeneration. Alzheimer's and Dementia, 10*(3), S242–S253. https://doi.org/10.1016/j.jalz.2014.04.003

Menon, D., Schwab, K., Wright, D., & Maas, A. (2010). Position statement: Definition of traumatic brain injury. *Archives of Physical Medicine and Rehabilitation, 91*(11), 1637–1640.

Munivenkatappa, A., Agrawal, A., Shulka, D., Kumaraswamy, D., & Devi, B. (2016). Traumatic brain injury: Does gender influence outcomes? *International Journal of Critical Illness & Injury Science, 6*(2), 70–73. https://dx.doi.org/10.4103%2F2229-5151.183024

Neal, C., Bell, R., Carmichael, J., DuBose, J., Grabo, D., Oh, J., Remick, K., Bailey, J., & Stockinger, T. (2018). Catastrophic non-survivable brain injury care – Role 2/3. *Military Medicine, 183*, 73–77. https://doi.org/10.1093/milmed/usy083

Okie, S. (2005). Traumatic brain injury in the war zone. *New England Journal of Medicine, 352*, 2043–2047. www.nejm.org/doi/full/10.1056/nejmp058102

Phillips, Y. (1986). Primary blast injuries. *Annals of Emergency Medicine, 15*(12), 1446–1450.

Ponsford, J. (2013). Mechanism, recovery and sequelae of traumatic brain injury: A foundation for the REAL approach. In J. Ponsford, S. Sloan, & P. Snow (Eds.), *Traumatic brain injury: Rehabilitation for everyday adaptive living* (2nd ed., pp. 1–33). Psychology Press.

Ponsford, J., Janzen, S., McIntyre, A., Bayley, M., Velikonja, D., & Tate, R. on behalf of the INCOG Expert Panel. (2014). INCOG recommendations for management of cognition following traumatic brain injury, part 1: Posttraumatic amnesia/delirium. *Journal of Head Trauma Rehabilitation, 29*(4), 307–320.

Taylor, C., Bell, J., Breiding, M., & Xu, L. (2017). Traumatic brain injury-related emergency department visits, hospitalizations, and deaths – United States, 2007 and 2013. *Morbidity and Mortality Weekly Report Surveillance Summaries, 66*(9), 1–16. http://dx.doi.org/10.15585/mmwr.ss6609a1

Teasdale, G., & Jennett, B. (1974). Assessment of coma and impaired consciousness: A practical scale. *Lancet, 304*, 81–84.

Theadom, A., Starkey, N., Dowell, T., Hume, P., Kahan, M., McPherson, K., & Feigin, V. (2014). Sports-related brain injury in the general population: An epidemiological study. *Journal of Science and Medicine in Sport, 17*(6), 591–596. https://doi.org/10.1016/j.jsams.2014.02.001

Winkler, E., Yue, J., Burke, J., Chan, A., Dhall, S., Berger, M., Manley, G., & Tarapore, P. (2016). Adult sports-related traumatic brain injury in United States trauma centers. *Neurosurgical Focus, 40*(4), 1–12. https://doi.org/10.3171/2016.1.FOCUS15613

3 Stages of Treatment

Case Study

The zesty broadcasting life of Patti Foster was instantly transformed from fully alive to fully dependent on June 18, 2002. She and three other ladies were in a Chevy Tahoe on their way to the final Bible study before the summer break. A semi (truck) a trailer full of cars slammed into their stopped sports utility vehicle (SUV). Patti was ejected from the back seat, through the stationary glass window, up into the air, falling and skidding across the highway, ultimately stopping in a lane of traffic. The following is her account of the accident and what stages of treatment she experienced from the moment of her injury to today.

Patti Foster – The Accident

After 6:45 p.m. on that blazing hot summer night, my traumatized brain and discombobulated body depended completely on medical life support to sustain me. Quicker than the tick of a clock, I instantaneously changed from having no need of medical treatment to 24/7 dependency on trauma care treatment. Stages of need followed the rhythm of my six-week coma, severe closed head injury, and multiple bodily injuries inside and out. As in many traumatic brain injury cases, the uncertainty of my survival and the choices of necessary medical treatment moved at its own pace. I was guided through five primary stages of treatment: acute hospital, inpatient rehabilitation, inpatient transitional rehabilitation, outpatient transitional rehabilitation, and discharge to home.

The initial stage of treatment was set into motion by the heroic efforts of the air ambulance medical team of East Texas Medical Center (ETMC) Air 1. The diagnosis of multi-trauma caused by the wreck resulted in the need for helicopter transport from the crash scene to a Level 1 trauma center. Trauma surgeons were contacted and provided details of my catastrophic injuries. They and the trauma nurses prepared for emergency treatment upon my arrival. At the scene, patient care records were completed. Details to indicate which treatments to

DOI: 10.4324/9781003301912-3

prescribe included fractures, abrasions, contusions, and lacerations of my ejected body. Wounds blanketed my head all over, but the right side appeared to have taken the worst impact. Blunt trauma showed its force on my chest, back, shoulders, both arms, hands, knees, ankle, and legs. Injuries required treatment to assist with airflow, breathing, circulation, along with the multiple damage to my torso and extremities that had glass and other unidentifiable debris from the highway embedded into my body.

Patti Foster – Acute Hospitalization

In the intensive care unit (ICU), I received continual care and monitoring while my life hung in the balance. My family was told that the first 24–48 hours were critical. I was given less than a 20% chance of survival. My family and friends and lots of radio listeners, dedicated prayer warriors, and innocent eyewitnesses needed care and treatment of some kind after such shocking news. They talked among themselves about what had happened. Their lives, too, had been affected by the traumatic wreck.

After more than five weeks of treatment in an acute hospital, my learning-to-live-again body was transported via ground ambulance to a leading inpatient rehabilitation facility in the nation – Baylor Institute for Rehabilitation (BIR) in downtown Dallas, Texas. The rehabilitation team addressed my agitation, right orbital fracture, contusions, abdominal and pelvic damage, right sacral and right superior and

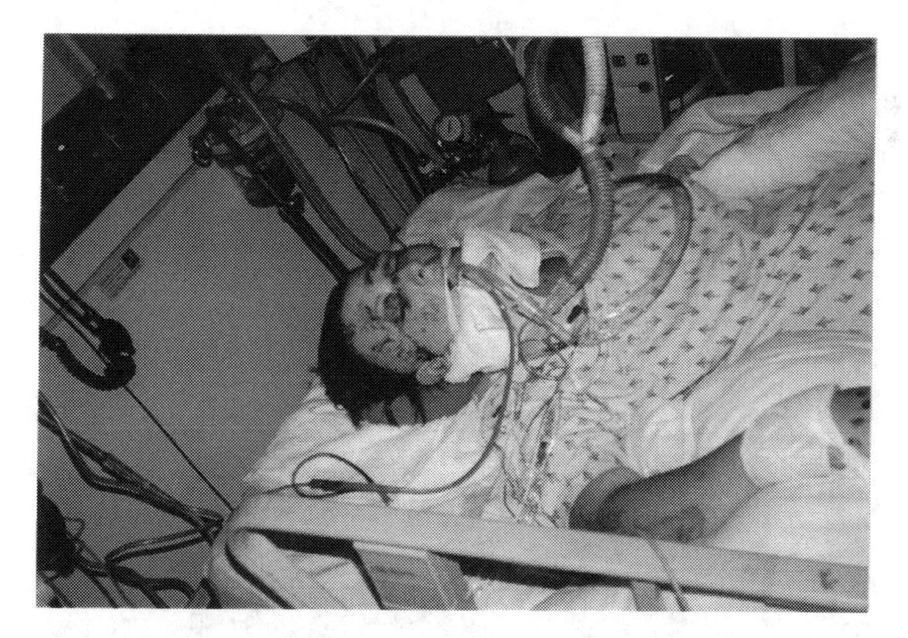

Figure 3.1 Patti Foster – acute hospital.

inferior cervical fractures, spine [*sic*] fractures, facial lacerations, bronchial problems, and multiple skin and tissue damage from my eyelids to the tips of my toes. Coma, dysphasia (a language disorder that makes it hard to communicate), and a percutaneous endoscopic gastrostomy (PEG) tube for nourishment were addressed. Rehabilitation activities began in the morning, with occupational therapy (OT) coming to my room to help me groom and get ready for the day. I spent each day with various therapists instructing [me] through rehabilitative treatments, including speech therapy (ST), physical therapy (PT), visual therapy, and cognitive therapy. An invaluable neuropsychologist oversaw my recovery and progress while at BIR.

Patti Foster – Inpatient Rehabilitation Hospital

The next stage of treatment was being admitted to an inpatient transitional rehabilitation facility. The treatment team recognized that my brain and body was [*sic*] only capable of low-level distractions and required high-level structure for me to progress. I was released from BIR and admitted to a facility a few hours north of Dallas. As my damaged brain continued to gain positive recovery, a moderate degree of assistance was needed. My insight was redeveloping, though at a lower level of perception and understanding as the transitional stage got underway. Treatment activities addressed impulsivity and balance. My strength needed developing so I could safely get up and down without assistance.

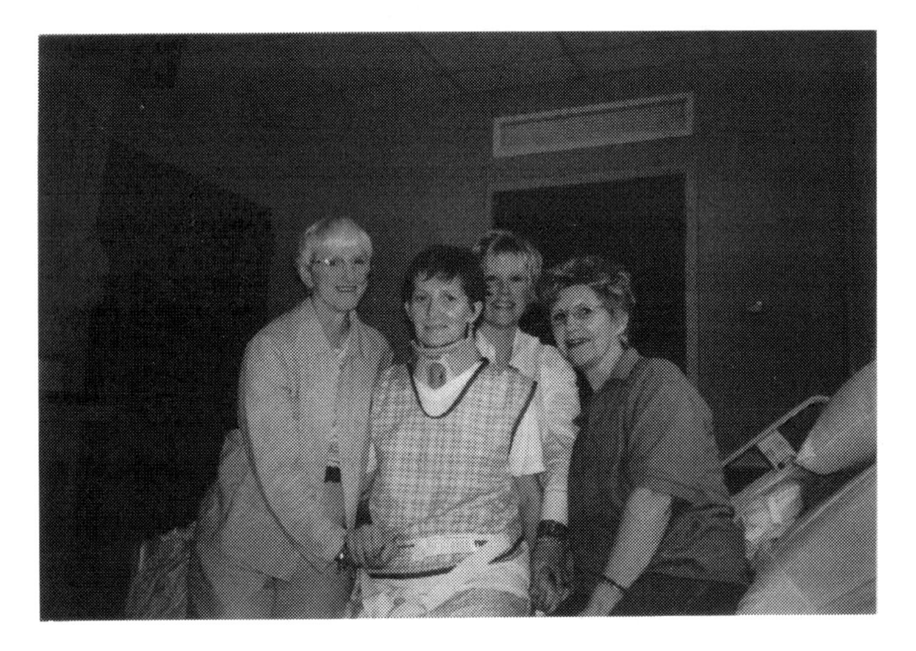

Figure 3.2 Patti Foster – inpatient rehabilitation.

Patti Foster – Inpatient Transitional Rehabilitation

As the medical team assessed my background and met with my family, they began to discover that the individual who filled that deeply injured brain and body had a "strong religious history." My family members were extremely supportive and clearly involved in the entire recovery process. My medical records reflected my cooperative attitude and hard work in relearning how to live again. Family conferences were scheduled monthly to discuss treatment and recovery updates. The treatment plan involved six hours per day, five days per week, with the goal that I would return to motivational speaking and broadcasting on the radio.

Preparations for optimal transitioning were being made for me to discharge to home. A case manager worked with [the] Texas Rehabilitation Commission to look for eligible services that might be a possibility for me. Returning to live with my family would most likely be appropriate since I would require some level of supervision. As work opportunities to speak and interview requests arrived, some degree of assistance would be helpful. Driving to and from events would be evaluated when indicated. My estimated discharge date was October 11, 2002. From that time, the transitional team planned my function level to require only supervision, my toleration (of distractions) level to move from low to moderate, and my need for structure to improve from a high need to a more moderate level required for a positive outcome. I was able to move home and attend outpatient transitional rehabilitation at the same facility.

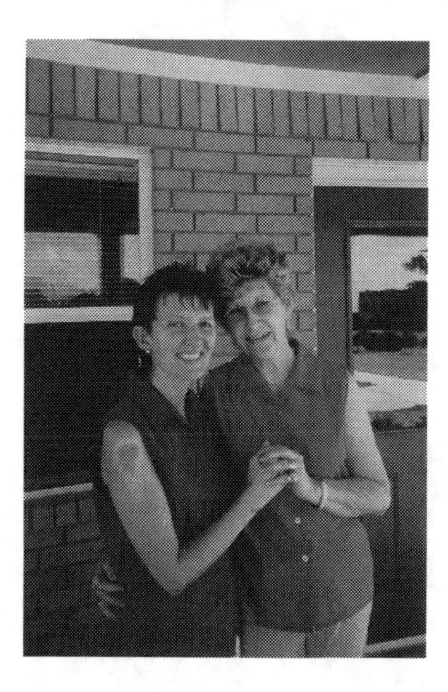

Figure 3.3 Patti and Judy Foster – transitional rehabilitation.

I want to acknowledge other treatments needed for recovery, such as counselors to address the mental healthiness and healing after a traumatic event. Christian counselors who have studied the short-term and long-term effects of brain injury and who spend time with a brain injury survivor can offer indescribable "medicine" and hope. They can awaken hope in the lives of brain injury survivors who are trying to thrive, caregivers and family members who want to help and be a healthy supporter [*sic*].

For me, the relationship I have with God through the Lord Jesus carries me steadfastly along this brain injury journey. Faith helps me persevere and not give up. Serving others and comforting them with the comfort and encouragement I myself have received helps take my attention off of my problems and fixes my attention on God and encourage[s] others along the way. Brain injury is consistently inconsistent, so please choose to lay hold of each moment.

For all the brain injured people who will ever read any of this book, don't give up! Lean in and persevere. As your life continues after brain injury, keep looking and searching for purpose [and] for your place in this world after things in your life have changed. And please, make the time to discover your motto for living. Mine is M.A.D. Now! (Make a Difference Now!). Search for yours and fully live it! Learning to cope can bring hope . . . your life has purpose.

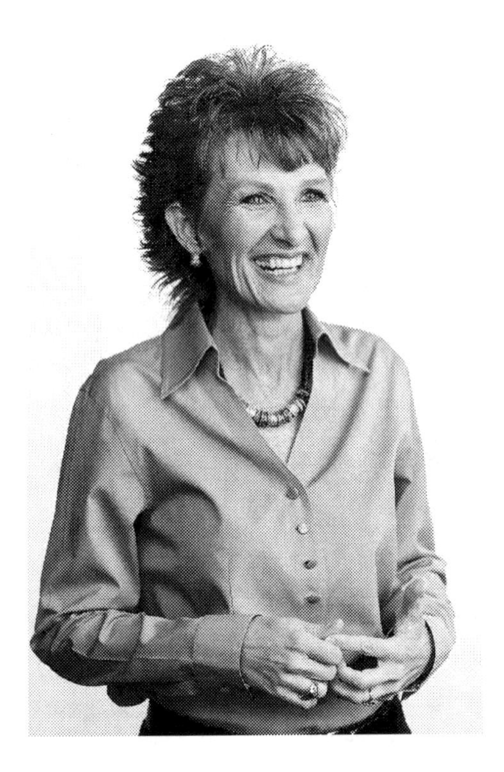

Figure 3.4 Patti Foster today.

Overview of Brain Injury Care

Each brain injury is unique, and each recovery path is different. However, there are similarities in the stages of treatment. Described next are the levels of treatment for a severe to moderate brain injury. The stages of treatment for a mild TBI may be less extensive. Normally, the initial stage of any brain injury requires emergent or urgent medical services. Distinctions for a lesser severity TBI will be noted throughout the text.

Emergent Care

Depending on the severity and the circumstances of the injury, the victim is taken to the nearest emergency department via car or ambulance. Medical treatment on the scene prepares the victim for transport, which includes stabilizing breathing and securing all wounds and fractures. Oxygen is provided because it is life-threatening for the brain to be deprived of oxygen for two or more minutes. Once at the hospital, a comprehensive examination of the body and brain is completed by the treatment team, which can include physicians, nurses, neurologists, neurosurgeons, maxillofacial surgeons, orthopedists, etc. Additionally, evaluations such as the Glasgow Coma Scale and the Rancho Los Amigos Scale of Cognitive Functioning (RLAS) are completed. The RLAS is utilized as the patient emerges from a coma and throughout the recovery process (Hagen et al., 1972). The original RLAS had eight scales. Two additional stages were later added to reflect the higher level of functioning in recovery (Lin & Wroten, 2021). A patient at level I is nonresponsive and requires total assistance. At level II, the patient still requires total assistance but exhibits generalized reflexes and gross body movements. At level III, the patient has localized responses, such as turning away from painful or auditory stimuli. The patient may respond to some members of the family but not to others. Level IV is characterized by a confused and agitated state of mind. This is when the patient attempts to remove restraints, has mood swings from euphoria to hostility, and is unable to cooperate with treatment. The patient at level V continues to require maximal assistance; although alert, s/he is not oriented to time, place, or person. The patient is unable to learn new information and does not have the ability for sustained attention or goal-directed, purposeful behavior. At level VI, the patient requires moderate assistance, vacillating between confusion and appropriateness. The patient can follow simple directions and has a vague recognition of others. S/he is unaware of his/her impairments, disabilities, or risky behavior. The patient at level VII is consistently oriented and able to perform simple activities of daily living. Minimal supervision is required at this level; however, the patient may overestimate his/her ability to function and can be oppositional or uncooperative and unaware of the feelings of others. Level VIII is characterized by purposeful and appropriate behavior. The patient can think about the consequences of his/her behavior and carry out learned tasks, but s/he is argumentative and easily agitated. Only stand-by assistance is required. At level

IX, the patient can move easily between tasks. S/he can use assistive memory devices and self-monitoring strategies. Assistance is by request. The final stage is level X. At this level, the patient can navigate between tasks, interact appropriately within a social setting, use compensatory strategies, and recognize the needs and feelings of others. Assistance is considered modified independent. Many survivors transition home at this level and may continue to require the modified independent level of assistance indefinitely.

Acute Hospitalization

Once the patient is stabilized, s/he is transferred to the intensive care unit. Treatment is adjusted hour by hour. The hospitalist or attending physician assesses and orders the various testing, medication, and monitoring for the patient. When the brain tissue is damaged (torn or bruised), it bleeds and swells, which creates pressure inside the inflexible skull. Intracranial pressure (ICP) can lead to secondary damage, so it is monitored closely. To measure the pressure, a surgeon may implant an ICP monitor into the skull just below the hairline. Continual monitoring of blood pressure, limiting fluids, and administering oxygen and medication maximize the recovery potential for the patient. Neuroimaging such as computerized tomography (CT), magnetic resonance imaging (MRI), functional magnetic resonance imaging (fMRI), positron emission tomography (PET), and single-photon emission computerized tomography (SPECT) scans may be ordered to determine the cerebral oxygen level, region cerebral blood flow, structural changes, and glucose metabolism (Snow & Ponsford, 2013). Electrophysiological and other technological examinations are ordered periodically to determine and treat the severity and complexity of the injuries. The length of stay at this level of treatment varies from 2–3 days to several weeks depending on the severity of the brain injury.

Disorders of Consciousness

Although a full discussion of the disorders of consciousness (DOC) is beyond the scope of this text, what follows is a brief synopsis of the history of DOC and terms that may be applicable to a person who has survived a severe brain injury, whether acquired or traumatic in nature. *Consciousness*, according to Posner and his co-workers (2007), is "the full state of awareness of the self and one's relationship to the environment." The term *coma* is generally understood as a pathological state of being unconscious. A coma usually "resolves within 2–4 weeks after the initial injury, and patients who remain unconscious by this point typically transition into either a vegetative state or minimally conscious state" (Whyte et al., 2019). In 1975, Jennett and Bond developed the Glasgow Outcome Scale (GOS), which described five broad categories of outcome for a severe TBI: death, persistent vegetative state (PVS), severe disability, moderate disability, and good recovery. The limitations of the scale warranted an extended version called the GOSE, developed by Jennett and colleagues in 1981. The GOSE divides severe disability, moderate disability, and good recovery in lower and upper extremities. In the mid-1990s, three position papers written by the American Academy of Neurology (1994), the American Congress of Rehabilitation Medicine (1995), and a multidisciplinary working group (Andrews, 1996) aimed to address the complexities of these severely injured patients. Unfortunately, these efforts did not simplify but rather complicated the diagnoses. As a result, the Aspen Neurobehavioral Workgroup (ANW) was formed to resolve the discrepancies of the first three position papers and deliver a consensus on terminology, diagnosis criteria, and management guidelines (Giacino & Whyte, 2005). The ANW made distinctions between the following conditions: coma, vegetative state (VS), minimally responsive state, and locked-in state (LIS). *Vegetative state* is "a state of unconsciousness in which the eyes are open but there is no awareness of self, others, or the environment" (Fins, 2015). Jennett (2002) believed that the qualifier "persistent" should be added if the patient was in a vegetative state for more than one month, and the qualifier "permanent" if longer than 12 months. Because some patients retain conscious awareness despite the loss of speech and volitional movement, efforts have made to replace the term "vegetative state" with "unresponsive wakefulness" (Laureys et al., 2010).

Minimally responsive state came to be known as *minimally conscious state* (MCS) and is considered a condition of severely altered consciousness characterized by minimal behavioral evidence of awareness of self or the environment. Giacino et al. (2002) stated that MCS "is one in which there is definite, albeit intermittent evidence of consciousness." Fins (2015) explains the difference between VS and MCS. He stated that, "MCS patients differentiate themselves from those in VS by virtue of behaviors that indicate an awareness of themselves or their external environment."

Finally, *locked-in state* (or syndrome) was first identified by Plum and Posner in 1966. LIS is "a condition in which there is essentially normal cognition but sparse motor output save for blinking and head movements" (Fins, 2015). Khanna et al. (2011) described LIS as a "disease process where the brain is fully functional while confined within a non-functional body." Bauer et al. (1979) subdivided LIS into three categories: (1) classical LIS describes total immobility except for eye blinking or vertical eye movement; (2) incomplete LIS exhibits remnants of voluntary movement; and (3) total LIS describes complete immobility, including eye movement, combined with preserved consciousness. It is hopeful that this short synopsis of DOC will shed light on and improve understanding of the complexities of severe brain injury.

Acute Inpatient Rehabilitation

The next stage of treatment is called acute inpatient rehabilitation. This can be a stand-alone facility or a unit in an acute-care hospital. The brain-injured patient's care includes an interdisciplinary team led by a physiatrist, also known as a physical medicine and rehabilitation physician (PM&R). The treatment team typically consists of a physical therapist, occupational therapist, speech therapist, recreational therapist, rehabilitation nurse, prosthetic or orthotic specialist, neuropsychologist, dietitian, and social worker. The patient has at least three hours of therapy a day for five to six days per week. The interdisciplinary team meets on a regular basis to assess the treatment goals and progress of the patient. These meetings may include family members as well as the patient, depending on his/her ability to comprehend and contribute to the discussion. In addition to ongoing assessment, the team develops a discharge plan, which may include stepping down to outpatient rehabilitation, to transitional care or home, or to an alternative living arrangement. The overall goal of acute inpatient rehabilitation is "to optimize a patient's quality of life and achieve maximal independent functioning" (Rosenberg et al., 2007).

Transitional Rehabilitation

Once the patient has met the treatment goals of the acute rehabilitation level of care, is medically stable, but is not ready to be in his/her home environment, s/he may be admitted to transitional rehabilitation (TR), also known as residential rehabilitation and/or post-acute rehabilitation. TR treatment programs are comprehensive, utilizing intensive physical, behavioral, and cognitive therapies, including counseling, development of compensatory skills, training in the use of assistive technology, and environmental modification. Additional therapists who may be involved at this stage of treatment are a vocational therapist, art therapist, music therapist, nutritionist, and a case manager, who is a supportive liaison between the patient and his/her funding source. The facility is community based and mimics real-world experiences, such as apartment-like rooms, group space, mock grocery store, and a vehicle. Transitional rehabilitation provides 24/7 supervision and is led by an interdisciplinary team as in acute rehabilitation facilities. In addition, they may offer community-based rehearsals to assist the patient to return to productive activities, driving, and improved quality of life. The real-life activities and group work help the patient gain self-awareness and develop social skills. Within the safety of the program, patients are allowed to make mistakes due to poor judgment or poor impulse control, enabling them to gain insight, fine-tune their goals, and enhance social cognition. The program focuses "on higher-level aspects of recovery and rehabilitation, including increased awareness of deficits, compensatory strategy building, and improved social and behavioral pragmatics" (Flashman & Barisa, 2019). Patients participate in at least six hours of therapy per day, which may include completing activities of daily functioning such as personal hygiene, laundry, and simple cooking. The length of stay for TR can vary from several weeks to several months. Before the patient is discharged from this stage of treatment, a family member is trained to assist and monitor medications, assist with ambulation, and ensure safety of his/her loved one. Additionally, a trained therapist will visit the patient's home to assess safety concerns and recommend needed modifications so that the home environment can safely accommodate the patient's residual disabilities. The transition to outpatient rehabilitation involves the patient visiting his/her home on a short outing of one to three hours, then a day away from the facility, and sometimes an extended weekend outing.

Outpatient Rehabilitation

The stages of treatment listed previously are recommended for moderate to severe brain injury survivors. Outpatient rehabilitation (subacute rehabilitation) can be recommended for all severities of brain injury. Normally, this is a structured group setting during the day and allows the survivor to return home at night. Also called day treatment or day rehabilitation, it is sometimes recommended in place of transitional rehabilitation, depending on the severity of the brain injury. The patient is transported to the outpatient facility for day treatment. The goal for this level of care is to assist the patient to reach his/her highest level of physical, functional, and cognitive independence. Therapies during day treatment focus on skills for increased independence and improved cognitive, behavioral, and emotional rehabilitation. Patients participate in various therapies for six hours each day. Services include cognitive therapy, physical, occupational, speech therapy, vision and vestibular therapy, education therapy, aquatic therapy, counseling and behavioral analysis, family education, group therapy, and community reintegration. Typically, the length of treatment at this level of care is 6–12 weeks. As in the other stages of treatment, the patient's care has the oversight of the medical treatment team assigned to his/her care.

Home Health Services

As the patient transitions to home from facility-based care, sometimes it is recommended that s/he participate in home health services. Although the various stages of treatment train various life skills, unfortunately some patients are unable to transfer those strategies to their home environment. Home health (HH) services provide rehabilitation through occupational, physical, and speech therapy in the home where the patient can re-learn adaptive skills. These services may also assist the patient to develop higher level motor, social, and cognitive skills to assist in the transition from home to the work environment. Other treatment strategies include social awareness, such as how to interact with others, money management, task initiation, and goal setting. Home health services often are recommended after the patient first discharges home but before outpatient therapy. Normally, after the patient has been home for a while, the family and the survivor can identify the deficits and areas that may need improvement. Employing home health services at that time helps to fine tune the recovery needs.

Vocational Rehabilitation

The working age brain injury survivor and his/her family hopes that s/he can return to work in some capacity. Vocational rehabilitation (VR) assesses the strengths and goals of the survivor, determines if s/he can return to his/her pre-injury job, capitalizes on residual skills, performs a functional vocational assessment, and establishes a selective placement and supportive employment plan. A functional vocational assessment is designed to determine the return-to-work options and the supports needed. Once the survivor of TBI is employed, the VR specialist (sometimes referred to as a job coach) may accompany the individual to his/her job and recommend accommodations needed for maximum success. Workplace support is divided into physical and cognitive/emotional assistance. Physical impairment assistance is meant to circumvent possible difficulties that may arise in the work environment, for example, modifying a workspace that ensures safety should the survivor experience dizziness or balance problems, addressing range of motion limitations, and utilizing assistive technology or adaptive equipment. Cognitive and emotional impairments include lack of awareness, impaired concentration/attention, memory impairment, and emotional and behavioral dysfunction. Accommodations in this category focus on developing emotional and behavioral self-regulation, increasing self-awareness, identifying triggers, modeling positive interactions, developing checklists/flow charts/memory helps, and counseling when the survivor experiences emotional distress (Wehman et al., 2011). Additionally, workspace accommodations need to address the decreased cognitive speed of the survivor and eliminate or reduce sensory input to alleviate or slow fatigue, for example, by providing a separate work area that allows for reduced lighting, reduced noise, and room temperature control. Shortened work hours and extended deadlines are also helpful. Specifically, it helps for the survivor to work during the morning hours before fatigue adversely affects performance. It may also be advantageous for the employer to allow time for the survivor to take mini breaks through the work shift. A VR will be able to educate the employer on the needs of someone who suffers from brain injury and how they can adjust for maximum success in the work experience.

Outpatient Counseling

The final stage of treatment is participation in outpatient counseling. The frequency and content of sessions are specific to each brain injury survivor and the family's needs. Generally, ongoing education, developing compensatory strategies, managing of emotional challenges, creating behavioral strategies, allowing for ambiguous grief, and creating a sense of purpose are the overall goals of outpatient counseling. The remainder of this text will address these issues individually from a brain injury survivor and family member perspective and offer Christian, faith-based, or nonspiritual counseling techniques for recovery.

Conclusion

This chapter began with the story of Patti Foster, a survivor of a severe TBI. She shared her experience of various levels of treatment. the stages of treatment from the onset of the injury through discharge to home were also identified. This chapter was meant to be an overview of the treatment and therapies associated with the recovery from brain injury. Depending on the severity of the injury, the patient may participate in acute hospitalization, inpatient rehabilitation, transitional rehabilitation, outpatient rehabilitation, and outpatient counseling. Ancillary services such as home health, vocational rehabilitation, and occupational, speech, and physical therapies are introduced as needed at different levels of recovery. The concept of disorders of consciousness was mentioned briefly in this chapter. The next chapter introduces the family experience of brain injury.

References

Andrews, K. (1996). International working party on the management of the vegetative state: Summary report. *Brain Injury*, *10*(11), 797–806.

Bauer, G., Gerstenbrand, F., & Rumpl, E. (1979). Varieties of locked in syndrome. *Journal of Neurology*, *221*, 77–91.

Fins, J. (2015). *Rights come to mind: Brain injury, ethics, and the struggle for consciousness*. Cambridge University Press.

Flashman, L., & Barisa, M. (2019). Neuropsychological assessment. In J. Silver, T. McAllister, & D. Arciniegas (Eds.), *Textbook of traumatic brain injury* (3rd ed., pp. 163–180). American Psychiatric Association Publishing.

Giacino, J., Ashwal, S., Childs, N. Cranford, R., Jennett, B., Katz, D., Kelly, J., Rosenberg, J., Whyte, J., Zafonte, D., & Zasler, N. (2002). The minimally conscious state: Definition and diagnostic criteria. *Neurology*, *58*(3), 349–353.

Giacino, J. & Whyte, J. (2005). The vegetative and minimally conscious states: Current knowledge and remaining questions. *Journal of Head Trauma Rehabilitation*, *20*(1), 30–50.

Hagen, C., Malkmus, D., & Durham, P. (1972). *Rancho Los Amigos Levels of Cognitive Functioning Scale*. Rancho Los Amigos Hospital.

Jennett, B., Snoek, J., Bond, M., & Brooks, N. (1981). Disability after severe head injury: Observations on the use of the Glasgow Outcome Scale. *Journal of Neurology, Neurosurgery & Psychiatry*, *44*(4), 285–293. https://doi.org/10.1136/jnnp.44.4.285

Jennett, B. (2002). Assessment of severity of head injury. *Journal of Neurology, Neurosurgery & Psychiatry*, *39*, 647–655.

Khanna, K., Verma, A., & Richard, B. (2011). "The locked-in-syndrome": Can it be unlocked? *Journal of Clinical Gerontology & Geriatrics 2*, 96–99.

Laureys, S., Celesia, G., Cohadon, F., Lavrijsen, León-Carrión, J., Sannita, W., Sazbon, L., Schmutzhard, E., von Wild, K., Zeman, A., Dolce, G., & European Task Force on Disorders of Consciousness (2010). Unresponsiveness wakefulness syndrome: A new name for the vegetative state or apallic syndrome. *BioMed Central Medicine*, *8*(68). https://doi.org/10.1186/1741-7015-8-68

Lin, K., & Wroten, M. (2021, August 30). *Rancho Los Amigos*. NCBI. www.ncbi.nlm.nih.gov/books/NBK448151/

Posner, J., Saper, C., Schiff, N., & Plum, J. (2007). *Plum and Posner's diagnosis of stupor and coma*. Contemporary Neurology.

Rosenberg, C., Simantov, J., & Patel, M. (2007). Physiatry and acquired brain injury. In J. Elbaum & D. Benson (Eds.), *Acquired brain injury: An integrative neuro-rehabilitation approach* (pp. 18–38). Springer.

Snow, P., & Ponsford, J. (2013). Assessing and managing impairment of consciousness following TBI. In J. Ponsford, S. Sloan, & P. Snow (Eds.), *Traumatic brain injury: Rehabilitation for everyday adaptive living* (2nd ed., pp. 34–65). Psychology Press.
Wehman, P., Goodwin, M., McNamee, S., & Targett, P. (2011). Return to work following traumatic brain injury. In F. Zollman (Ed.), *Manual of traumatic brain injury management* (pp. 450–456). Demos Medical Publishing, LLC.
Whyte, J., Bergin, M., & Giacino, J. (2019). Disorders of consciousness. In J. Silver, T. McAllister, & D. Arciniegas (Eds.), *Textbook of traumatic brain injury* (3rd ed., pp. 201–216). American Psychiatric Association Publishing.

4 Family Experience of a Loved One With Brain Injury

Case Study

When news of Patti's crash spread, friends and family came to the hospital. Because Patti was a radio personality, the facility was inundated with people from all over the area. Hospital staff had to relocate the visitors to a different floor of the hospital to accommodate such an influx of people. Hundreds of listeners, family members, and friends prayed for Patti and the three other ladies injured in the traffic crash. Shock, disbelief, and confusion were just a few of the feelings experienced by the family, which included her parents, her brother, and his wife. The first 48 hours were critical. Patti was in a coma with her life hanging in the balance. Thankfully, after several days, even though she was still in a coma, Patti's condition stabilized.

Judy, Patti's mom and main caregiver, did not understand at first why her daughter had to be transferred to another facility because she was receiving such great care. The treatment team at the acute care hospital did not fully communicate the extent of Patti's injuries or what the rehabilitation process would entail. Judy thought that her daughter would recover in the hospital and then be discharged home. An intensive care nurse was the one who explained that Patti would need rehabilitation to help her recover from her traumatic brain injury. Because they were from a small community, the closest rehabilitation facility was two hours away. Patti's mom had to make arrangements with her employer and her family so that she could be with her daughter throughout the next stage of treatment. When Patti was transferred by land ambulance, the receiving hospital's nurse explained to Judy what to expect. Patti would be at this hospital as she began to wake from her coma and relearn the basics of living. Judy never left the facility. She slept, washed her clothes, etc. at the hospital. They let her stay and treat it just like it was her home too. She was with Patti during most of her therapies. After several weeks, another transition of care was recommended. Due to the severity of Patti's TBI, she would need to be transferred to an transitional rehabilitation hospital . . . an hour outside of the metroplex. Now Judy would be three hours from her daughter. Once Patti was admitted, Judy was not allowed to stay overnight as she was at the previous hospital. The separation, the unknown, and the fear of not being with her daughter

DOI: 10.4324/9781003301912-4

were extremely difficult for Judy. Patti's brain began to improve, and her injuries were healing. The treatment team at this facility helped Patti with "activities of daily living," from performing personal hygiene to speaking in front of others. Before the wreck, Patti was a radio personality and a motivational speaker. After a few weeks at this level of rehabilitation, Patti was able to return to her home. Judy was given limited information about what to expect from the deficits caused by the brain injury, much less how to handle them. Many in the community were also unaware of how to approach Patti or how to help her mom. Friends visited less often. Judy and Patti both relied on their faith in God to help them. After some time, Patti was able to begin speaking at church events. She was not yet able to drive herself, so her mom accompanied her to all of her speaking engagements. When Patti was ready, she returned to the hospital in the metroplex for outpatient therapy to learn to drive again and receive her license.

Patti and her family continue to deal with the long-term effects of brain injury. It has been years since the wreck, and Patti has learned to cope with the cognitive and emotional deficits from the TBI. Although she looks the same as before the injury, Patti is different. She struggles with hypersensitivity including light and auditory sensitivity, unusually instant agitation and being easily distracted, anger, balance, headaches, and fatigue. However, she and her family continue to depend on God's faithfulness and to celebrate how He has given Patti new opportunities to inspire and encourage other brain injury survivors around the world to persevere. She has written several books and volunteers with several non-profit organizations, spreading encouragement and hope.

Impact of Brain Injury on the Family

Brain injury has two victims: the individual and the family. Both are at the mercy of slow recovery, difficult emotional and physical deficits, limited resources, uninformed friends, a frustrating medical system, an unsure future, and a capsized life. The emotional and practical impacts on the family system are often unrecognized and untreated. The brain injury becomes an extra "person" or factor in the family system. Therefore, the family, their loved one, and the treatment team are all at the mercy of the brain injury, its effects, and its slow process of improvement. The family or caregiver (used synonymously) is rarely equipped to manage or cope with the far-reaching effects of brain injury (Sabella & Suchan, 2019). Winslade (1998) stated that once the brain-injured individual peaks in his/her recovery, the burden of care falls on the family, but the "challenge is greater than most families can cope with." Rotondi et al. (2007) explained that family members often "provide emotional support, instrumental and financial assistance, housing, and advocacy; facilitate rehabilitation and communications with providers; and identify needed services and service providers." Therefore, the family can both directly and indirectly influence the outcome of their loved one's recovery. The close relation between the well-being of a caregiver and that of a care receiver "suggests that assessment of caregiver impact, and subsequent management of caregiver health and burden, should be an integral part of the healthcare services provided for persons with TBI, as well as a key measure of their effectiveness" (Rotondi et al., 2007). Research has found that caring for a person with a TBI has an adverse effect on the caregiver or care partner and can extend for years post-injury. Therefore, education and preparation of family members for the long-term effects of brain injury should be an integral part of the discharge planning process.

Impact on Relationships

Researchers have postulated that a spouse "faces greater challenges and obstacles than a parent, including the intangibles of living with a person who is likely to be different from the individual he or she married" (Koberstein, 2010). Some researchers have found that at least one-half of marriages will end in divorce. However, Arango-Lasprilla et al.'s (2008) study across two years post-injury found that only 15% of marriages ended in separation or divorce. They did find that a younger patient (36 years or younger) had approximately four times greater chance of marital instability than an older patient (57 years or older). Additionally, they found that the severity of TBI affected marital stability: the less severe the TBI, the greater the marital stability. Gender was found to influence marital stability such that the "odds of being unstably married were 1.95-times higher for males with TBI than for females with TBI" (Arango-Lasprilla et al., 2008). Kreutzer et al. (2007) found that marital stability was associated with injury severity. They reported that a longer period of unconsciousness was associated with a greater likelihood of divorce. A protective factor was duration of the relationship. Couples in "surviving relationships were married nearly three times longer than those in relationships that dissolved" (Kreutzer et al., 2007). Although many have found that most marriages do not survive a brain injury, there are some researchers who have discovered factors that contribute to a positive outcome. Koberstein (2010) suggested that reduced self-appraised burden; belief in self-efficacy and empowerment; self-reliance; reciprocal communication and effective relations between the injured person and his/her family; and caring, trustworthy, and uplifting social support contributed to a more positive outcome for marriage.

Chronister and Chan (2006) suggested parents may experience a higher level of social support than spouses, who experience a greater role change than parents. The tragedy of brain injury "ripples out to touch husbands and wives, parents and children" (Winslade, 1998). Parents face unique challenges, such as an extended parenthood phase. It is essential that family members and care partners be an integral part of the treatment team for brain injury survivors, because a supportive family is one of the best indicators for achieving the most adaptive outcome possible for a person with a brain injury (Ruff & Chester, 2014).

Families coping with brain injury have a higher incidence of anxiety disorders, mood disorders, and social adjustment issues (Hanks et al., 2007). One of the stressors on the family is the difficulty that the survivor of TBI has in modulating his/her emotional reactions, resulting in outbursts, flattened affect, or lability. Additionally, the patient may exhibit an inability to self-monitor or self-correct, thereby creating a deterioration in social graces and social judgment. The complexity of deficits such as self-centeredness, irresponsibility, lack of self-direction, self-control, or common sense inevitably leads to social dependency (Lezak, 1986).

Family Needs

Family needs are a crucial topic of study. Often, families and survivors feel that "they are moving from crisis to crisis, and simply reacting as new situations arise, with inadequate anticipation, planning, or guidance" (Rotondi, 2007). Researchers have documented that, during the acute and post-acute stages of recovery, the family needs clear communication about the patient's condition and prognosis. They also need information about the patient's treatment and resources. Additionally, emotional support, respite, and maintenance of hope are needed (Kolakowsky-Hayner et al., 2001). Various studies show that the needs of the family tend to change over time. Kolakowsky-Hayner et al. (2001) found that four years post-injury, the need for professional support was met the least often. They recommended that caregivers would greatly benefit from community- or web-based support groups, long-term case management services, ongoing family therapy, and assistance with household and family responsibilities. The Rotondi et al. (2007) study recognized needs already identified in other studies, such as the following: an understanding of injuries, treatments, and consequences; emotional and mental health of the person who experienced the TBI; financial assistance; guidance on how to care for the patient and facilitate recovery; family emotional and mental health as they learn to adapt to changes; finding and evaluating providers; quality of services and support from professionals; employer support; community integration; having a support group as well as support from family and friends; respite services; care coordination; and life planning. In sum, the authors recommended that providers offer honest, understandable, and complete information about the injuries, their sequelae, and the prognosis for recovery; answer questions and provide emotional and psychological support; provide anticipatory guidance; teach stress management, problem-solving, and behavioral management techniques; facilitate life planning; and emphasize community integration. Sadly, these are often overlooked in the acute care phase of treatment. Therefore, it is necessary for counselors to revisit these issues and assist the family in making accommodations in the home environment.

Stages of Recovery

In 1992, Rape, Bush, and Slavin published a critique of the developmental stage models of recovery experienced by families of survivors of TBI that had been put forth by various researchers (Lezak, 1986; Spanbock, 1987; Henry et al., 1985; Groveman & Brown, 1985). Spanbock (1987) and Henry et al.

(1985) postulated that the first stage is initial shock when the family experiences denial, helplessness, confusion, frustration, and anger. Stages two, three, five, and six were described by Lezak (1986), Spanbock (1987), Henry et al. (1985), and Groveman & Brown (1985). The second stage is emotional relief, denial, and unrealistic expectations. The expectations include the denial of deficits, believing that the loved one will return to premorbid functioning and thereby experience a problem-free future. The third stage is acknowledgment of permanent deficits and emotional turmoil. The family perceives the patient as uncooperative, unmotivated, and self-centered, while the family is bewildered, anxious, and depressed. Families miss the premorbid functioning of their loved one and attribute the family disruption to his/her behavior problems. The family begins to acknowledge the permanent deficits, which can create feelings of despair, withdrawal, depression, and entrapment. Bargaining is the fourth stage described only in Groveman & Brown (1985) model whereby there is a regression to unrealistic demands and the expectation of a return to premorbid functioning. Mourning and working through loss are the fifth stage. The family acknowledges the permanent deficits, misses the premorbid functioning, and mourns their loss. The final stage is acceptance and restructuring, which involves a redefining and restructuring of the family relationships and roles. My experience is that families normally seek counseling between the second and fifth stages.

Lezak (1986) offered suggestions for psychologists as they work with families through the various stages of recovery. Initially, counseling is little more than establishing the groundwork for future sessions. The clinician may help the family observe changes in their loved one's behavior and demeanor. The second stage provides an opportunity for the psychologist to assist the family in identifying behaviors that cause problems, understanding the natural symptoms of brain injury, and discovering what they can do to mitigate or navigate the deficits. The third stage is when conflicts within the family system become more pronounced. The psychologist can speak frankly about the irreversible effects of brain injury and create a constructive disengagement from the past. If the family can learn coping strategies, this will help to reduce friction and to improve interactions with the survivor of TBI. For example, the family can learn to avert the outbursts of a loved one by introducing a benign topic or activity. In stage four, according to Lezak (1986), many families can

> engage in the explicit task of learning to see the patient as different from before – a person whom they neither raised nor chose, who cannot be satisfied or give satisfaction in any adult emotional sense, and whose unpleasant behavior should not be taken personally.

The fifth stage is when the psychologist gives the family permission to mourn and reassures them that their feelings are completely normal considering their current challenges. The final stage allows the psychologist to assist in reinterpretation of the relationships within the family. At this phase of treatment, the clinician's greatest usefulness may be in connecting the family to community resources. Lezak (1986) underlines the necessity for psychologists to convey the naturalness of both the problem behaviors and the family's reaction to them. Understanding the concept of naturalness may relieve the family and their loved one of self-doubt, guilt, and fear. It may be helpful to identify the brain injury as another member of the family. I have found that reframing is helpful for accepting the reality of the injury and its effects on the family system.

Caregiver Burden

Caregiver burden or the distress caused by caregiving is multifaceted. It has been "characterized as a multidimensional response to various stressors associated with caregiving, affecting the social, psychological, physical, and emotional aspects" (Manskow et al., 2015). Marsh et al. (2002) found that caregivers most often reported less time for themselves, increased anxiety, changes in sleep pattern, less privacy, changes in their financial situation, and changes in their relationships. Increased physical illness, less time for themselves, and a change in employment were reported as causing the most stress on the caregiver. Additionally, the survivors' behaviors that involved emotional control were reported as causing a great degree of distress to their caregivers. Due to the severity of the brain injury, Marsh et al. (2002) suggest that caregiving for a loved one with a severe TBI impacts not only close family relationships but also extended family relationships. Winslade (1998) stated that spouses of individuals with a brain injury

> are often torn between guilt about wanting to abandon the injured partner and resentment at having to sacrifice so much of their own lives and satisfactions to care for someone who often doesn't appreciate the burdens undertaken on his or her behalf.

Hanks et al. (2007) suggest reappraising caregiver burden in more positive terms because it is likely to positively affect caregiver well-being. Their study supported previous research that indicated "social support reduces the adverse influence of stress associated with caregiving." They also found that "caregivers who report high social support also report more positive appraisals of the burden, relationship satisfaction, and mastery experienced in caregiving." Last, the caregiver's ideology "was the sole aspect of caregiving unrelated to perceived social support." Ideology, specifically one's moral or traditional ideas about caregiving, was most firmly held among caregivers "who focused on proactive problem solving and who disregarded the intensity of demands and the support available to assist them in meeting the challenges of caregiving." There is evidence that caregiving involves both positive and negative feelings and can provide opportunities for growth, challenge, and satisfaction (Chronister & Chan, 2006). Norma, the wife of a TBI survivor, stated that her full-time care of her husband was an extension of the love she had had for him since they were both young children. She shared that she had loved him from childhood and would love him through his homegoing.

Chronister and Chan (2006) studied the various coping methods utilized by caregivers of a brain-injured loved one. They document that Chwalisz (1996) found that coping was positively related to perceived stress, with problem-focused coping negatively linked to perceived stress and emotion-focused coping (acceptance, positive reappraisal, spiritual support) positively linked to perceived stress (Chronister & Chan, 2006). Active coping, denial and emotional disengagement, avoidance, self-control, confrontation, and accepting responsibility contributed to higher levels of stress (Kosciulek, 1994). The ability to frame caregiving in a positive light decreased caregiver burden and reduced stress.

Chronister and Chan (2006) reported a gender difference in coping responses. Female caregivers tend to use both emotion-focused and problem-focused coping efforts more frequently than males. They also experience a higher burden and higher satisfaction from their caregiving. Problem-focused coping (active coping and planning) assists the caregiver to feel some aspect of control over the outcome of the situation and to hope for change by seeking services, problem-solving, and helping the loved one move toward independence. However, the outcome of the efforts may not always meet the expectations, thereby leading to frustration, helplessness, increased burden, and distress. Avoidant coping (denial and mental and behavioral disengagement) was positively linked to burden and negatively linked to mastery, meaning those who utilized avoidant coping felt a greater burden and experienced less of a feeling of mastery. Finally, Chronister and Chan found that emotion-focused coping "was linked to satisfaction, suggesting that emotional acceptance and reappraisal may benefit TBI caregivers because of the limited control they have over the outcome of the situation" (Chronister & Chan, 2006). They found that time post-injury was negatively linked to problem-focused coping. In the early stages of recovery, caregivers utilized coping strategies that focused on creating a plan to solve a problem. In the latter stages of recovery, emotion-focused coping proved more useful because caregivers had adjusted to the enduring nature of the injury and the changes in their lives. The caregivers perceived and benefited from desirable factors of the caregiving experience and thereby felt more satisfaction.

Physical and Financial Impacts

The experiences of the family are different depending on the stage of recovery of their loved one. Families experience "a high incidence of psychosomatic disorders, and increased consumption of psychotropic medication and alcohol" (Marsh et al., 2002). Initially, families may experience shock, denial, disbelief, and anger immediately after an injury (Mathis, 1984). Anxiety and stress are common after the initial injury, although these issues may continue for the first year of recovery. Marsh et al. (2002) suggested that physical disabilities are seen as more socially acceptable, especially for the first six months of recovery. However, at one year post-injury, the caregiver and survivor realize that improvement of physical impairment is less likely, which can cause greater distress.

There is limited empirical evidence on how financial hardship is associated with caregiving. However, there are issues of changing family employment and income, high medical costs, and unknown financial future for the injured loved one. Sabella and Suchan (2019) suggested that financial burden be given more attention as part of holistic support strategies. Their study found that effective financial support "may include benefits planning assistance, financial literacy instruction, or employment supports for the individual with TBI and family members." Connecting families to state- and community-funded resources helps to alleviate the financial burden of brain injury recovery.

Psychosocial Impact

Psychosocial health encompasses the mental, emotional, social, and spiritual aspects of life. The most disabling dysfunction after brain injury is the psychosocial deficits (Rosenthal & Bond, 1990). The changes in personality and social behavior that can occur can limit the individual's capacity for a successful return to work, independent living, and the rehabilitation of social relationships with peers and family members (Kosciulek, 1994). Once the survivor's physical impairments are stabilized, the focus shifts to the cognitive and behavioral deficits of brain injury.

Social isolation has been recognized as one of the most distressing aspects of caregiving. Unfortunately, research demonstrates that the lack of social contact is a permanent feature of the long-term outcome of severe TBI (Marsh, 1999). Social support is "a broad concept that could include all of the social resources available to individuals, including interpersonal ties, professional support, and health resources" (Manskow et al., 2015). In Scandinavia, Manskow et al. (2015) found that one-half of the caregivers in their study "reported medium or high caregiver burden, and that the strongest predictors for a high burden were more severe disability in patients and poor quantity and quality of the caregiver's social network." Douglas and Spellacy (2000) found a positive association between social support and distress, perceived neuropsychological deficits, family functioning, and well-being. They believed that education about the consequences of TBI among the community, including professionals, doctors, teachers, and/or ministers, assisted in lowering the social isolation of caregivers. Chronister and Chan (2006) reported that increased social support was linked to lower burden and better quality of life for caregivers. Tomberg et al. (2005) found that the availability of potential supporters "contributes to positive adjustment and problem solving and provides a buffer against the effect of stress." They also stated that it is essential for the brain-injured person to develop community-based support and counseling to integrate the social aspect with occupational activity. The caregiver's perception of available practical support, such as help with transportation, housesitting, and availability of emotional support with someone with whom to talk to and share common situations, contributed to a more positive caregiving experience. Feelings of loneliness and decreased contact with close friends were significant factors in increased caregiver burden (Manskow et al., 2015). Loneliness may partly reflect "an experience of being different from other individuals because of the TBI specific experience, in addition to actual social isolation" (Manskow et al., 2015). Social organizations, churches, and religious organizations can play a key role in alleviating the social burden and isolation of families and survivors.

Interventions

Support for caregivers who may report depression, marital stress, financial loss, social isolation, anxiety, and somatic symptoms involves helping them with problem-solving abilities. Various researchers have identified cognitive-behavioral therapy, education, family therapy, and support groups as means of mitigating the adverse effects of caregiving (Marsh et al., 2002). Powell et al. (2016) found that problem-solving interventions have been shown to decrease the distress of family caregivers and has been associated with improvement in the care recipient's depression, social function, and behavior. The problem-solving approach used in this study began with acknowledgment of the brain injury, which assists the caregiver in accepting that there will be significant challenges coupled with believing that s/he can meet those challenges. Second, there is a goal-setting portion that implements specific strategies. In Powell et al.'s (2016) study, the caregivers were educated on topics such as physical and medical issues; strategies for coping with emotional and behavioral challenges; strategies for coping with changes in thinking and communication; how to manage activities at home; how to be a caregiver; the emotional issues of caregiving; strategies for taking care of one's own health; social support; and strategies for getting things done. The results of their study showed that caregivers experienced more positive outcomes, especially their emotional well-being. They felt more equipped to care for themselves and their loved one with a brain injury. Leach et al. (1994) observed that effective problem-solving and coping strategies used by family members were inversely associated with depression experienced by a survivor.

Interventions based on hope, stress management, and coping skills are indicated to be important in couple and family work in the recovery and rehabilitation processes (Manskow et al., 2015). Marital intervention "has the potential to remediate declining relationship quality, relieve couples' psychological distress, and diminish caregiver burden" (Kreutzer et al., 2020). The Therapeutic Couples Intervention (TCI) adapted from the Brain Injury Family Intervention (BIFI) designed by Emilie Godwin, Jeffrey Kreutzer, and Jennifer Marwitz (Kreutzer et al., 2020) addresses issues commonly confronting couples after brain injury. The structured treatment program is designed to enhance the quality and stability of relationships by education, skill-building, and psychological support. TCI (supported by the tenets of cognitive-behavioral therapy) relies heavily on specific therapy techniques such as normalization, reframing, empathic reflection, and validation. Kreutzer et al. (2020) found that caregivers for survivors of all severities of TBI were assisted by TCI, with the partners of individuals with moderate to severe injuries benefiting more than the partners of individuals with mild injuries.

Dausch and Saliman (2009) utilized family-focused therapy (FFT) as an intervention for the rehabilitation of veterans with traumatic brain injury. They stated that the impact on the families of veterans is complicated because the families of returning TBI survivors are already strained due to the deployment. Additionally, the family system must adapt to markers of recovery for the brain-injured loved one. For example, if their loved one shows the ability to manage his/her finances, the family must accommodate this area of recovery by creating oversight while allowing him/her to use this skill. This is one of the ultimate goals of therapy and is consistently trained/advocated by PT/OT/ST in rehabilitation. FFT suggests that "maximizing healthy family functioning and facilitating periodic renegotiations of what is adaptive for the family may ameliorate the extent of which the individual with TBI is disabled" (Dausch & Saliman, 2009). The model focuses on enhancing the family system through providing information about TBI and the rehabilitation process, as well as skills training to improve relational functioning. It moves beyond simply the relief of symptoms and offers problem-solving and communication skills that cultivate a collaborative partnership between the survivor of TBI, the family, the community, and the healthcare team. The goal is to improve the survivor's "ability to participate in meaningful life activities and valued roles" (Dausch & Saliman, 2009). The FFT intervention is consistent with the goals of auxiliary rehabilitation such as physical, speech, and occupational therapies.

In 1991, McCubbin and McCubbin created the Resiliency Model of Family Stress, Adjustment, and Adaptation. They defined family coping as a "specific effort, covert or overt, by which an individual family member or the family as a whole attempts to reduce or manage a demand on the family" (Kosciulek, 1994). Family adaptation is the "outcome of family efforts to bring a new level of harmony, balance and coherence to the family system after a crisis" (McCubbin & McCubbin, 1991). Kosciulek et al. (1993) used this model as a framework for working with the families of survivors of head injury. One of the results of Kosciulek's (1994) study found that "the family that views a head injury as a manageable family challenge will most likely adapt more successfully than a family that views an injury as catastrophic." Coping strategies such as taking a break from caregiving, openly expressing emotions, and attending church services were recommended for managing stress. Additionally, breaking down problems into manageable steps assisted families in managing tension. Family adaptation appears to be strongly influenced by "family efforts to maintain a positive attitude and realistic outlook toward the family and head injury situation" (Kosciulek, 1994).

Lezak (1986) recommended clarification of the terms clinicians use to explain the recovery process. She pointed out that when clinicians use the word "recovery," they mean "improvement," but laypeople equate "recovery" with "return to normal." Religious people "may take survival to be a sign of divine intervention, and their expectations for complete recovery may withstand the test of reality for months or even years" (Lezak, 1986). The patient's familiar appearance may cause the family to respond to him/her in the same way as they did the pre-injury person, that is, the person they remember instead of who s/he currently is. Clarifying expectations regarding recovery and potential will help the family adjust their view of their loved one and correct the normal (although incorrect) perception that s/he is the same as before the injury. It is more helpful for the family to observe their loved one develop skills and personality in the same way they would watch a newborn become his/her own person.

Family Navigator

Powell et al. (2016) suggested that assistance for caregivers must move beyond symptom management and resource identification to a mentor-focused approach. Telephonic training as well as face-to-face interaction is recommended. Educational material may be presented in various formats such as short videos or written in a less dense, more graphic-oriented way to improve efficiency. Social support has been shown to act as a cognitive moderator of positive outcomes for caregivers (Hanks et al., 2007). Recommendations for effective caregiving support include providing caregivers with skills to deal with the behavioral problems that they feel they can routinely invoke; encouraging active problem-solving strategies versus focusing on emotional toll; and providing social support and educating families to facilitate realistic expectations about caregiving (Hanks et al., 2007).

In 2016, Patti Foster, a survivor of TBI, created the Family Navigator (FN) program. The goal of the FN program is to connect the family of a person with a newly diagnosed brain injury with a trained volunteer who is either an experienced caregiver of a brain-injured person or a survivor of brain injury. The volunteer will partner with the family from the onset of a brain injury diagnosis throughout the rehabilitation process and the return to the community, or until the family communicates that the FN is no longer needed. The role of the FN is to support, educate, and encourage the family as their loved one moves through the various stages of treatment and improvement. The volunteer must successfully complete the training program, which addresses listening skills, effective mentoring, interpersonal and communication skills, resource development, successful caregiving, ethics, and coping strategies. Like a peer mentoring program, the FN will work alongside an individual and family, offering his/her experience, listening, answering questions and offering suggestions, researching resources, assisting with transitions of care, assisting with coping with the challenges of brain injury deficits, and educating. In summary, the FN will help family members and survivors to navigate through the medical and rehabilitative processes and the transition to home and work environments. By sharing their experiences and real-world insights, FNs will assist families of brain injury survivors to thrive in their recovery. To date, the FN program, in collaboration with Hope After Brain Injury is being implemented within the state of Texas and is expanding throughout the United States.

Conclusion

Brain injury affects the entire family for the whole of the rest of their lives. Unfortunately, the burden of care for the survivor falls on the family, who are typically unequipped to manage the effects of the injury. This chapter discussed the physical, psychosocial, and financial impacts of brain injury on the family. Additionally, the stages of recovery as they coincide with the emotional reactions from the caregiver were addressed. Commonly understood interventions including problem-solving and emotional coping were described. The Family Navigator program was explained. The next chapter details the brain, its functions, and the deficits associated with the areas of the brain affected by injury.

References

Arango-Lasprilla, J., Ketchum, J., Dezfulian, T., Kreutzer, J., O'Neil-Pirozzi, T., Hammond, F., & Jha, A. (2008). Predictors of marital stability 2 years following traumatic brain injury. *Brain Injury, 22*, 565–574. https://doi.org/10.1080/02699050802172004

Chronister, J., & Chan, F. (2006). A stress process model of caregiving for individuals with traumatic brain injury. *Rehabilitation Psychology, 51*(3), 190–201.

Chwalisz, K. (1996). The perceived stress model of caregiver burden: Evidence from spouses of persons with brain injuries. *Rehabilitation Psychology, 41*(2), 91–114.

Dausch, B., & Saliman, S. (2009). Use of family-focused therapy in rehabilitation for veterans with traumatic brain injury. *Rehabilitation Psychology, 54*(3), 279–287. https://doi.org/10.1037/a0016809

Douglas, J., & Spellacy, F. (2000). Correlates of depression in adults with severe traumatic brain injury and their carers. *Brain Injury, 14*, 71–88.

Groveman, A., & Brown, E. (1985). Family therapy with closed head injured patients: Utilizing Kubler-Ross' model. *Family Systems Medicine, 3*, 440–446.

Hanks, R., Rapport, L., & Vangel, S. (2007). Caregiving appraisal after traumatic brain injury: The effects of functional status, coping style, social support and family functioning. *NeuroRehabilitation, 22*, 43–52.

Henry, P., Knippa, J., & Golden, C. (1985). A systems model for therapy with brain-injured adults and their families. *Family Systems Medicine, 3*, 427–429.

Koberstein, E. (2010). Family life. In P. Klonoff (Ed.), *Psychotherapy after brain injury: Principles and techniques* (pp. 150–170). Guilford Press.

Kolakowsky-Hayner, S., Miner, K., & Kreutzer, J. (2001). Long-term life quality and family needs after traumatic brain injury. *Journal of Head Trauma Rehabilitation, 16*(4), 374–385.

Kosciulek, J. (1994). Relationship of family coping with head injury to family adaptation. *Rehabilitation Psychology, 39*(4), 215–229.

Kosciulek, J., McCubbin, M., & McCubbin, H. (1993). A theoretical framework for family adaptation to head injury. *Journal of Rehabilitation, 59*(3), 40–45.

Kreutzer, J., Marwitz, J., Hsu, N., Williams, K., & Riddick, A. (2007). Marital stability after brain injury: An investigation and analysis. *NeuroRehabilitation, 22*, 53–59.

Kreutzer, J., Marwitz, J., Sima, A., Graham, K., Hsu, N., Mills, A., & Lukow, H. (2020). Evaluation of a brief, skill-building, supportive, and educational intervention for couples after brain injury. *Journal of Head Trauma Rehabilitation, 35*(3), 175–186. https://doi.org/10.1097/HTR.0000000000000519

Leach, L., Frank, D., Bouman, D., & Farmer, J. (1994). Family functioning, social support, and depression after traumatic brain injury. *Brain Injury, 8*, 599–606.

Lezak, M. (1986). Psychological implications of traumatic brain damage for the patient's family. *Rehabilitation Psychology, 31*(4), 241–250.

Manskow, U., Sigurdardottir, S., Røe, C., Andelic, N., Skandsen, T., Damsgård, E., Elmståhl, S., & Anke, A. (2015). Factors affecting caregiver burden 1 year after severe traumatic brain injury: A prospective nationwide multicenter study. *Journal of Head Trauma Rehabilitation, 30*(6), 411–423.

Marsh, N. (1999). Social skill deficits following traumatic brain injury: Assessment and treatment. In S. McDonald, L. Togher, & C. Code (Eds.), *Communication disorders following traumatic brain injury* (pp. 175–210). Psychology Press.

Marsh, N., Kersel, D., Havill, J., & Sleigh, J. (2002). Caregiver burden during the year following severe traumatic brain injury. *Journal of Clinical and Experimental Neuropsychology, 24*(4), 434–447.

Mathis, M. (1984). Personal needs of family members of critically ill patients with and without acute brain injury. *Journal of Neurosurgical Nursing, 16*, 36–44.

McCubbin, M., & McCubbin, H. (1991). Family stress theory and assessment: The resiliency model of family stress, adjustment, and adaptation. In H. McCubbin & A. Thompson (Eds.), *Family assessment inventories for research and practice* (pp. 3–32). University of Wisconsin-Madison.

Powell, J., Fraser, R., Brockway, J., Temkin, N., & Bell, K. (2016). A telehealth approach to caregiver self-management following traumatic brain injury: A randomized controlled trial. *Journal of Head Trauma Rehabilitation, 31*(3), 180–190.

Rape, R., Bush, J., & Slavin, L. (1992). Toward a conceptualization of the family's adaptation to a member's head injury: A critique of developmental stage models. *Rehabilitation Psychology 37*(1), 3–21.

Rosenthal, M., & Bond, M. (1990). Behavioral and psychiatric sequelae. In M. Rosenthal, E. Griffith, M. Bond, & J. Miller (Eds.), *Rehabilitation of the adult and child with traumatic brain injury* (2nd ed., pp. 179–182). Davis.

Rotondi, A., Sinkule, J., Balzer, K., Harris, J., & Moldovan, R. (2007). A qualitative needs assessment of persons who have experienced traumatic brain injury and their primary caregivers. *Journal of Head Trauma Rehabilitation, 22*(1), 14–25.

Ruff, R., & Chester, S. (2014). *Effective psychotherapy for individuals with brain injury*. Guilford Press.

Sabella, S., & Suchan, C. (2019). The contribution of social support, professional support, and financial hardship to family caregiver life satisfaction after traumatic brain injury. *Journal of Head Trauma Rehabilitation, 34*(4), 233–240.

Spanbock, P. D. (1987). Understanding head injury from a family's perspective. *Cognitive Rehabilitation, 5*, 12–14.

Tomberg, T., Toomela, A., Pulver, A., & Tikk, A. (2005). Coping strategies, social support, life orientation and health-related quality of life following traumatic brain injury. *Brain Injury, 19*(14), 1181–1190. https://doi.org/10.1080/02699050500150153

Winslade, W. (1998). *Confronting traumatic brain injury: Devastation, hope, and healing*. Yale University Press.

5 Brain Anatomy, Functions, and Deficits

*I would like to extend my great appreciation to Dr. Karen Brewer-Mixon who reviewed and offered expert content for this chapter.

Brain Anatomy

A typical human is born with approximately 100 billion neurons in the brain (Sakai, 2020). The complexity, speed, and sophistication of the brain functions rely on the 100 trillion or so interconnections between these neurons to govern every thought and activity required within the body, as well as every processing and perceiving function within the environment. Even after an injury, neuroscientists have discovered that nerve cells can "regenerate when prompted by certain nerve growth factors . . . traumatic brain injury itself appears to switch on genes that may trigger the release of healing chemicals" (Winslade, 1998). The science behind neuroplasticity is a field of study that holds promise for the recovery potential of the human brain. The brain and the spinal cord comprise the central nervous system of the body. The brainstem, cerebrum, cerebellum, and cranial nerves make up the brain. Some of the deeper structures of the brain are the hypothalamus, pituitary gland, amygdala, and hippocampus. Although a full explanation is beyond the scope of this book, what follows is an overview of the brain's anatomy and functions, followed by the potential deficits associated with injury to each portion of the brain.

Brainstem

The brainstem connects the cerebrum to the spinal cord and is composed of three sections: the midbrain, the pons, and the medulla oblongata. It serves as a relay station, passing messages back and forth between the spinal cord (via the peripheral nervous system) and the brain. The midbrain facilitates various functions such as ocular motion, hearing, movement, coordination, calculation of responses, and environmental changes. The pons connects the midbrain to the medulla and is the origin of four of the 12 cranial nerves. It regulates tear production, chewing, blinking, focusing of vision, and balance, and it coordinates eye and facial movement as well as controls the vestibulocochlear nerve

DOI: 10.4324/9781003301912-5

responsible for hearing. The medulla oblongata is at the bottom of the brainstem and connects to the spinal cord. It is essential to survival, regulating many bodily activities such as heart rhythm, respiration, blood flow, and oxygen and carbon dioxide levels. The medulla also assists with reflexive and involuntary movements such as sneezing, vomiting, coughing, and swallowing. The reticular activating system works within all three sections of the brainstem to regulate sleep, wakefulness, and attention to the environment.

Studies of brain injury (Kim, 2012) have indicated that the incidence of traumatic brainstem injury during a brain injury varies between 8.8% (Hashimoto et al., 1993) and 52% (Firsching et al., 2002). A head injury prognosis becomes much graver if the brainstem is involved. When the brainstem is injured, it can result in paralysis, respiratory problems, swallowing problems (dysphagia), coma, locked-in syndrome (patient is cognitively aware but can only move his/her eyes), or death. Milder consequences of brainstem injury include difficulties managing body temperature, sleep dysfunction, nausea, balance issues, and slurred speech.

Cerebrum

The cerebrum (also called the forebrain) is the largest part of the brain, accounting for two-thirds of total brain weight. It comprises gray matter (the cerebral cortex) at the outer layer and white matter at its center. The gray matter of the brain consists of unmyelinated axons branching off neurons, the dendrites of neurons, and glia. Glial cells provide support and nutrition to the neurons and maintain cell homeostasis. White matter consists of a brain cell's axons that are covered in myelin, a multilayer of protein and lipids that helps the parts of the brain communicate efficiently by facilitating rapid signal transmission in the nervous system.

The cerebrum is divided into two hemispheres connected by the corpus callosum, through which areas on the two sides of the brain communicate with each other. In terms of motor functioning, the right side of the brain controls the left side of the body, and the left side of the brain controls the right side of the body. Each hemisphere is further divided into four lobes: frontal, temporal, parietal, and occipital.

Frontal Lobes

The frontal lobes are the largest region of the brain, constituting almost one-third of the human brain. Cicerone et al. (2006) divided the executive functions of the frontal lobes into four categories: executive cognitive functions, behavioral self-regulatory functions, activation regulating functions, and metacognitive processes. The executive cognitive functions are high-level cognitive functions that control and direct the lower-level, more automated functions. These higher-level functions include planning, monitoring one's behavior and the environment, activating, switching, and inhibiting. Generally, executive cognitive functions plan any goal-directed and purposeful action. They involve working memory, which has limited memory capacity, and very short-term memory storage. Burke et al. (1991) described executive functioning as determining whether and how the person can complete a task. Cognitive impairment usually implies a specific functional deficit, while executive functioning impairment affects all aspects of one's daily life (Burke et al., 1991).

Behavioral self-regulatory function is self-control as it pertains to emotional processing and stimulus-reward associations. Self-control involves "having the discipline to stay on task despite distractions and completing a task despite temptations to give up, to move on to more interesting work, or to have a good time instead" (Diamond, 2013). Emotional processing is important to creating successful social interactions. Social cognition refers to the ability to process social information and perceive social cues, such as facial expressions, body language, and other nonverbal forms of communication (Westerhof-Evers et al., 2019). Activation regulating function provides initiation and energizing behavior to make decisions appropriate for the situation. Lezak (1988) believed that executive functions included the ability to formulate goals, develop plans, carry out those plans, and effectively monitor and regulate goal-directed performance. On the other hand, executive functioning impairments are "manifested by emotional lability, irritability, rigidity, apathy, carelessness, poor judgment and inappropriate social behavior" (Burke et al., 1991).

Metacognitive processes (thinking about thinking) integrate executive cognitive functions with self-regulatory behavior. These processes are involved with "personality, social cognition, autonoetic consciousness, and self-awareness as reflected by the accuracy of evaluating one's own abilities and behavior in relation to objective performance and reports by others" (Cicerone et al., 2006). Self-appraisal, a feature of metacognition, is one's ability to personally reflect on one's own knowledge, abilities, and motivation. Self-management, another key feature of metacognition, involves one's mental processes that help to problem-solve, adjust, review results, and make necessary revisions (Papleontiou-louca, 2003).

Cicerone et al. (2006) stated that "the effects of TBI on executive functioning are dynamic in the sense that these abilities are impaired immediately after injury and recover at a variable rate depending on severity of focal and diffuse effects." Focal effects pertain to specific areas of the brain affected, while diffuse effects involve damage spread throughout several areas of the brain. Deficits in the frontal lobe affect perception, gross and fine motor abilities, information processing, naming and word-finding, attention, reasoning, and judgment and may result in maladaptive behaviors such as impulsivity, aggression, and hostility (Kois et al., 2018). Survivors of TBI with frontal lobe damage may have difficulty with complex activities such as following the plot on a television show, carrying on a lengthy conversation, remembering to wear a coat in cold weather, speaking at a normal pace, or recognizing social cues needed to participate in social discourse. Frontal lobe injury creates issues with sequencing, inflexible thinking, perseveration, personality changes, inability to focus on a task, apathy, lack of empathy, egocentricity, and anosognosia (lack of awareness or lack of insight about one's impairment). Additionally, the personality of a person with a frontal lobe brain injury may be altered.

Temporal Lobes

The temporal lobes are the second largest lobes of the human brain. They are associated with eight cognitive domains: language production, receptive language, hearing, episodic memory, phonological knowledge (the ability to attach meaning to sounds), semantic knowledge (long-established knowledge about objects, facts, and word meaning), social knowledge (processing, thinking about, remembering, and attending to the self and others in a social situation), and visual memory (Patel et al., 2021). The temporal lobes are essential for processing memory, language, and some aspects of emotion. Wernicke's area, located in the posterior part of the left temporal lobe, was named after German neurologist Carl Wernicke, who first related language deficits to the temporal lobe of the brain.

Disturbances in the temporal lobes can lead to a range of emotional and behavioral changes, from slight issues up to aggressive or homicidal tendencies. Difficulty with facial recognition (prosopagnosia), poor regulation of eating and sexual behavior, and impaired language function are associated with temporal lobe damage. Wernicke's aphasia impairs the ability to grasp the meaning of spoken words including their own words which are nonsensical, though fluent. If the anterior parts of the temporal lobe are damaged, then nearby Broca's area is likely to be damaged, which creates a struggle to produce words. Sometimes there is the issue of conduction aphasia in which the connections between Wernicke's area and Broca's area are disrupted. If this happens, the person can understand speech and usually talk fairly well but cannot repeat what others say and cannot read aloud. Wernicke's aphasia is sometimes called "fluent aphasia." Persons with this disability are able to speak using correct sentences with normal rate. However, often the words that are said do not make sense or the sentences are peppered with nonexistent or irrelevant words. Another aspect of an injured temporal lobe can be persistent talking. Two dysfunctions also found in temporal lobe damage are alexia (inability to read or comprehend written language), or agraphia (impairment or loss of the ability to write).

Parietal Lobes

Located near the posterior and top of the brain, the parietal lobes are responsible for processing and integrating somatosensory information from the body, including taste, smell, hearing, sight, and touch. This also includes pain, temperature, and sense of body movement and position (proprioception). These lobes allow one to recognize objects in the environment from touch, such as feeling for one's keys in a purse or recognizing bed covers in the dark. As they integrate sensory input, they construct a spatial coordinate system to represent the external environment.

Damage to the parietal lobes may result in Gerstmann's syndrome, which is a cognitive disorder characterized by difficulties in the ability to write (dysgraphia), to perform mathematics (dyscalculia), to distinguish between right and left (left-right disorientation), and to name, move, or touch one's fingers when directed to do so (finger agnosia). Balint's syndrome is a rare condition that results from bilateral damage to the parietal lobes. Parvathaneni and Das (2021) described this syndrome as characterized by optic ataxia (lack of coordination for reaching visual goals), oculomotor apraxia (deficit in voluntary, purposeful eye movement), and simultagnosia (inability to perceive more than one object at a time). Difficulty drawing objects, spatial disorientation, navigation difficulties, lack of awareness of body parts and surrounding space, and inability to focus visual attention are all aspects of parietal lobe injury. One survivor of TBI with parietal lobe damage would routinely miss a loop when putting on his belt. He stated that he knew it was there but could not make his brain direct his hands. Another survivor wore clothes that were not weather appropriate because she could not determine hot or cold outside temperatures. Parietal lobe damage can also cause hemispatial neglect or hemineglect in which the person is not aware of or is unable to attend to one side of his/her field of vision. The person cannot attend to the source of sounds on the side opposite where the brain injury occurred. Left neglect is most common. Audry, a brain injury survivor with damage to the right hemisphere of the brain, cannot find food on the left side of her plate. She does not notice people on the left side of her room. She may run into a door with her left shoulder, not realizing she has not cleared the doorway.

Occipital Lobes

The occipital lobes are the smallest of the four brain lobes. They sit under the occipital bone in the posterior part of the skull where the head meets the neck. The main function of the occipital lobes is to process visual information, including depth perception, color determination, distance perception, and object and face recognition (also a function of the right temporal and frontal lobes).

Damage to the occipital lobe may cause optic aphasia, which is characterized by difficulty identifying visually presented stimuli such as pictures, objects, or colors (Mårtensson et al., 2014). Cortical blindness can result from occipital lobe injury and has the distinct characteristic of visual anosognosia. An individual with visual anosognosia believes that s/he can see and confabulates visual perceptions, despite the loss of sight. This phenomenon is called Anton's syndrome, named after Austrian neurologist and psychiatrist Gabriel Anton. Other occipital lobe injury issues include visual hallucinations, visual illusions, visual field cuts (loss of peripheral vision, loss half of the visual field; may also be found with damage to parietal and temporal lobes), and color agnosia (inability to recognize color).

Cerebellum

Referred to as the "little brain," the cerebellum sits below the temporal and occipital lobes of the brain. This fist-sized portion of the brain plays a significant role in motor movement regulation and balance control. It coordinates gait, maintains posture, and controls muscle tone and voluntary muscle activity (Jimsheleishvilli & Dididze, 2021). Although it accounts for only 10% of brain volume, it contains 50% of the brain's neurons and approximately 80% of the central nervous system's neurons (Azevedo et al., 2009). Recent studies have suggested that the cerebellum may also play a role in cognition (including memory), behavior, and psychiatric illness (Rapoport et al., 2000). Damage to the cerebellum produces uncoordinated movements. Additionally, issues such as "language disorder, impairment of visuospatial cognition, impairment of executive function and mood changes are reported in association with tumours and vascular disorder of the cerebellum" (Maeshima & Osawa, 2009). Other difficulties associated with damage to the cerebellum are poor coordination, tremors, inability to perform rapid movements, and inability to judge distance and when to stop.

Cranial Nerves

The cranial nerves are a set of 12 pairs of nerves that originate on the underside of the brain and send electrical signals between the brain and different parts of the neck, head, and torso. There are sensory cranial nerves and motor cranial nerves. Each nerve pair splits to serve each side of the brain and body. The cranial nerves are identified with a Roman numeral and are ordered by location from front to back. The olfactory nerve is closest to the front of one's head and thereby designated first. The names and functions of each cranial nerve pair follow (Brennan, 2021; Seladi-Schulman, 2019).

- I Olfactory – The olfactory nerve transmits sensory information to the brain about smells.
- II Optic – The optic nerve carries visual information from the retina to the brain.
- III Oculomotor – The oculomotor nerve controls most of the eye movements, as well as the way in which the pupil constricts and the ability to keep the eyelid open.
- IV Trochlear – The trochlear nerve controls upward, downward, and outward eye movements.
- V Trigeminal – The trigeminal nerve is the largest of the cranial nerves and has both sensory and motor functions. The three branches of this nerve are the ophthalmic (sends sensory information from the upper part of the face, including forehead, scalp, and upper eyelids), maxillary (sends sensory information from the middle part of the face, including cheeks, upper lip, and nasal cavity), and mandibular nerves (sends sensory and motor information from the ears, lower lip, chin, and jaw).

VI Abducens – The abducens nerve is associated with lateral eye movement.

VII Facial – The facial nerve serves sensory and motor functions. It controls the muscles responsible for generating facial expressions. It also provides taste to two-thirds of the mouth and tongue.

VIII Vestibulocochlear – The vestibulocochlear nerve transmits sound and balance information from the inner ear to the brain. The cochlear portion detects vibrations of sound based on the sound's loudness and pitch and generates those impulses to the cochlear nerve. The vestibular portion tracks linear and rotational movements of the head and transmits the information to the vestibular nerve, thereby adjusting balance and equilibrium.

IX Glossopharyngeal – The glossopharyngeal nerve serves motor and sensory functions. It sends sensory information from the sinuses, the back of the throat (tonsils), parts of the inner ear, and the back part of the tongue. It also provides a sense of taste on the back of part of the tongue. Last, it stimulates voluntary movement of the muscle in the back of the throat called the stylopharyngeus.

X Vagus – The vagus nerve serves sensory and motor functions and has a longer pathway than all of the other cranial nerves, extending from the brain to the abdomen. It is responsible for sweating, heart rate, muscle movements in the mouth, and making sure the vocal cords are open for breathing and closed for speaking and swallowing. The vagus nerve communicates sensory information from the ear canal and parts of the throat. It stimulates the muscles of organs in the chest and trunk, including those that move food through the digestive tract (peristalsis).

XI Accessory – The accessory nerve controls the muscles in the neck. It allows one to rotate, flex, and extend muscles in the neck and shoulders.

XII Hypoglossal – The hypoglossal nerve controls tongue movements for speech, eating, and swallowing.

Damage to the cranial nerves can be temporary or permanent. The most common signs of cranial nerve disorders are pain in different regions of the body, tingling sensations in the neck or extremities, tactile sensitivity, vertigo, hearing loss, olfactory loss, inability to control facial expressions, problems with speech, trouble swallowing, and weakened or paralyzed muscles (Brennan, 2021). Different types of cranial neuropathies are Bell's palsy (drooping of one side of the face), microvascular cranial nerve palsy (double vision and eyesight problems), third nerve palsy (eyelid sags or droops, double vision, difficulty moving the eye, pupil is larger than normal), fourth nerve palsy (abnormal turning of the eye), or sixth nerve palsy (abnormal movement of the eye and double vision).

Hypothalamus

The hypothalamus rests at the base of the brain between the thalamus and the pituitary gland and is about the size of an almond. It receives messages from various parts of the brain, releasing and inhibiting hormones that act on the pituitary gland to direct the functions of the thyroid gland, adrenal glands, kidneys, musculoskeletal system, and reproductive organs (Shahid et al., 2021). The hypothalamus is the link between the endocrine and nervous systems and affects processes such as heart rate, blood pressure, body temperature, fluid and electrolyte balance, appetite, body weight, glandular secretions of the stomach and intestines, and sleep cycles (Sargis, 2021).

Damage to the hypothalamus include poor and excessive heat dissipation and body temperature fluctuations. There may also be a dysfunction in the circadian rhythm or unusual increases or decreases in appetite (Sahid et al., 2021). Brain injury survivors with damage to this region of the brain may have difficulty managing their appetite, eating too much because of the brain's inability to trigger the desire to stop eating or "feel full" at a meal. They also may experience greater thirst, loss of interest in activities, headaches, blood pressure fluctuations, and fatigue.

Pituitary Gland

The pituitary, sometimes referred to as the "master gland," is a pea-sized gland that sits at the base of the brain and controls the function of most other endocrine glands. Divided into two parts, the pituitary gland has an anterior and a posterior lobe. The anterior lobe accounts for 80% of the gland's weight. The hypothalamus controls the anterior lobe by releasing hormones through the connecting vessels. It controls the posterior lobe through nerve impulses. The anterior lobe releases six major hormones: adrenocorticotropic hormone (stimulates the adrenal glands to produce cortisol and other hormones), follicle-stimulating and luteinizing hormones, growth hormone, prolactin, and thyroid-stimulating hormone. The posterior lobe produces vasopressin and oxytocin (Carmichael, 2021).

Pituitary dysfunction occurs in approximately 20–40% of patients diagnosed with moderate to severe traumatic brain injury (Sav et al., 2019). Some of the diagnoses resulting from pituitary malfunction are growth hormone deficiency, hypogonadism (reduction in or absence of hormone secretion in testes or ovaries), hypothyroidism (underactive thyroid), hypocortisolism (adrenal insufficiency), and diabetes insipidus (an uncommon disorder that causes an imbalance of fluid in the body). Sav et al. (2019) stated that "anterior pituitary hormone deficiency has been shown to cause morbidity and increase mortality in TBI patients." A study from Greece recognized the importance of a comprehensive assessment of anterior pituitary function in the early and post-acute phases of treatment because "ongoing hormone deficiencies may adversely affect the recovery and quality of life of these patients" (Ntali & Tsagarakis, 2019).

Amygdala

The amygdala is a small, almond-shaped structure deep within the anterior temporal lobe and is the integrative center for emotions, emotional behavior, and motivation (Wright, 2020). It has extensive connections with other corticolimbic regions of affective processing (Leung et al., 2018). It is the front part of the limbic system and is loosely considered the brain's security guard, because it is constantly aware of stimuli in the environment. The limbic system is also called the "primitive brain" because of its role in survival instincts such as hunger, motivation, sex drive, mood, pain, pleasure, appetite, and memory (Anand & Dhikav, 2012). A common understanding is that the amygdala activates the "fight or flight" response when a person perceives a threat. The amygdala is involved in both pleasurable and fearful emotional learning and is where emotion and memory are combined. It is commonly thought "to form the core of a neural system for processing fearful and threatening stimuli including detection of threat and activation of appropriate fear-related behaviors in response to threatening or dangerous stimuli" (Baxter & Croxson, 2012). It is the engine that drives the neural coding of emotional identity in the limbic system and therefore connects to the emotional response to pain. Research suggests that the processing of potentially frightening things in the environment can reach the amygdala before one is consciously aware that there is anything to be afraid of; this is because frightening stimuli travel through the amygdala before they reach the cerebral cortex. Researchers have reported that "the amygdala is important for the detection and recognition of emotional facial expressions, for the processing of social information more generally, for advantageous complex decision-making, for taking the perspective of others, and for fear conditioning" (Rubin et al., 2014).

The amygdala is the part of the brain that wakes one up from a deep sleep due to the sound of a strange noise. As one realizes that the noise is an ice maker and nothing to be fearful of, the brain relaxes and allows one to return to sleep. Conversely, a damaged amygdala impairs the learning of new fear associations, the experience of fear, and the preferential processing of threatening environmental stimuli (Weber et al., 2016). Damage to the amygdala results in difficulty in recognizing emotional facial expressions, especially fearful ones (Baxter & Croxson, 2012). Research suggests that

> structural and functional abnormalities of this brain region are associated with affective pathologies . . . depression, post-traumatic stress disorders, anxiety, and dysfunctional retrieval of emotional autobiographical memories in older people. Additionally, bilateral amygdala damage disrupts affective but not cognitive empathy.
>
> (Leung et al., 2018)

Cognitive empathy refers to the ability to recognize and understand someone's mental state, while affective empathy refers to the ability to share the feelings of others.

Hippocampus

Hippocampus means "seahorse" in Greek and was named thus because this part of the brain looks like a seahorse. Its S-shaped structure is located deep within the temporal lobe and is part of the limbic system. The hippocampus is an area vital for memory, learning, and mood. While the amygdala is specialized for the input and processing of emotion, the hippocampus is essential for declarative memory, which is the storage of facts, and episodic memory, which is the storage of personal events like birthdays, anniversaries, etc. It is the back portion of the limbic system and 100 times smaller in volume than the cerebral cortex (Anand & Dhikav, 2012). The hippocampus is a critical structure involved in spatial and nonspatial memory. The amygdala and hippocampal complex "govern two independent memory systems that interact when emotion meets memory" (Yang & Wang, 2017). The hippocampus is "vital for learning, memory, and spatial navigation" (Anand & Dhikav, 2012). It can also affect motor behavior. The amygdala and hippocampus have reciprocal connections and, thus, influence one another. Rubin et al. (2014) stated that the hippocampus plays "a critical role by forming and reconstructing relational memory representations that underlie flexible cognition and social behavior." They also found that the hippocampus "is critical for performance in complex and ecologically valid situations that unfold over time and involve dynamically binding together various pieces of information."

Head trauma is associated with atrophy of the hippocampus (Anand & Dhikav, 2012). Other conditions that cause hippocampal volume reduction are Alzheimer's disease, schizophrenia, epilepsy, hypertension, and Cushing's disease. An insult to the hippocampus can render an individual

> unable to integrate knowledge during a complex task, use specific details to plan a future event, track the status of a social interaction over time, and, more generally, reach outside the contents of their current experience, or exhibit broader disruptions of everyday life.
>
> (Rubin et al., 2014)

Hippocampal damage may result in the inability to form and retain new memories. Rubin et al. (2014) stated that, because the hippocampus is integral to forming and reconstructing relational memory, damage to this area would lead to "inflexible and maladaptive behavior when such behavior places high demands on the generation, recombination, and flexible use of information." Individuals with a hippocampal insult may have difficulty recognizing and navigating social and potentially dangerous social situations because of an impaired ability to judge others' character and limited social discourse.

Conclusion

This chapter gave an overview of several functions of the brain as well as how those areas are affected by damage. Similarities in function and interrelationships between the regions of the brain were noted. The central nervous system (the spinal cord and the brain) and the peripheral nervous system (nerves outside the spinal cord and brain) communicate with the body for optimum functioning. When any of those areas are damaged due to brain injury, a myriad of issues and conditions result. This chapter gave a glimpse of many of these deficits associated with brain trauma.

References

Anand, K., & Dhikav, V. (2012). Hippocampus in health and disease: An overview. *Annals of Indian Academy of Neurology, 15*(4), 239–246. https://doi.org/10.4103/0972-2327.104323

Azevedo, F., Carvalho, L., Grinberg, L., Farfel, J., Ferretti, R., Leite, R., Filho, W., Lent, R., & Herculano-Houzel, S. (2009). Equal numbers of neuronal and nonneuronal cells make the human brain an isometrically scaled-up primate brain. *Journal of Comparative Neurology, 513*, 532–541. https://doi.org/10.1002/cne.21974

Baxter, M., & Croxson, P. (2012). Facing the role of the amygdala in emotional information processing. *Proceedings of the National Academy of Sciences, 109*(52), 21180–21181. https://doi.org/10.1073/pnas.1219167110

Brennan, D. (2021, January 4). *What are the 12 cranial nerves and their function?* MedicineNet. www.medicinenet.com/what_are_the_12_cranial_nerves_and_their_function/article.htm

Burke, W., Zencius, A., Wesolowski, M., & Doubleday, F. (1991). Improving executive function disorders in brain-injured clients. *Brain Injury, 5*(3), 241–252.

Carmichael, J. (2021, March). *Overview of the pituitary gland.* Merck Manual Consumer Version. www.merckmanuals.com/home/hormonal-and-metabolic-disorders/pituitary-gland-disorders/overview-of-the-pituitary-gland

Cicerone, K., Levin, H., Malec, J., Stuss, D., & Whyte, J. (2006). Cognitive rehabilitation interventions for executive function: Moving from bench to bedside in patients with traumatic brain injury. *Journal of Cognitive Neuroscience, 18*(7), 1212–1222.

Diamond, A. (2013). Executive functions. *Annual Review of Psychology, 64*, 135–168. www.annualreviews.org/doi/10.1146/annurev-psych-113011-143750

Firsching, R., Woischneck, D., Klein, S., Ludwig, K., & Döhring, W. (2002). Brainstem lesions after head injury. *Neurological Research, 24*, 145–146.

Hashimoto, T., Nakamura, N., Richard, K., & Frowein, R. (1993). Primary brainstem lesions caused by closed head injuries. *Neurosurgical Review, 16*, 291–298.

Jimsheleishvilli, J., & Dididze, M. (2021, July 31). *Neuroanatomy, cerebellum. StatsPearls Publishing.* www.ncbi.nlm.nih.gov/books/NBK538167/

Kim, J. (2012). The prognostic factors related to traumatic brainstem injury. *Journal of Korean Neurosurgical Society, 51*(1), 24–30. https://doi.org/10.3340/jkns.2012.51.1.24

Kois, L., Blakely, S., Gardner, B., McNally, M., Johnson, J., Hamer, R., & Elbogen, E. (2018). Neuropsychological correlates of self-reported impulsivity and informant-reported maladaptive behaviour among veterans with posttraumatic stress disorder and traumatic brain injury history. *Brain Injury, 32*(12), 1484–1491.

Leung, M., Lau, W., Chan, C., Wong, S., Fung, A., & Lee, T. (2018). Meditation-induced neuroplastic changes in amygdala activity during negative affective processing. *Social Neuroscience, 13*(3), 277–288. https://doi.org/10.1080/17470919.2017.1311939

Lezak, M. (1988). *Neuropsychological assessment* (2nd ed.). Oxford University Press.

Maeshima, S., & Osawa, A. (2009). Stroke rehabilitation in a patient with cerebellar cognitive affective syndrome. *Brain Injury, 21*(8), 877–883. https://doi.org/10.1080/02699050701504273

Mårtensson, F., Roll, M., Lindgren, M., Apt, P., & Horne, M. (2014). Sensory-specific anomic aphasia following left occipital lesions: Data from free oral descriptions of concrete word meanings. *Neurocase, 20*(2), 192–207. https://doi.org/10.1080/13554794.2012.741258

Ntali, G., & Tsagarakis, S. (2019). Traumatic brain injury induced neuroendocrine changes: Acute hormonal changes of anterior pituitary function. *Pituitary, 22*(3), 283–295. https://doi.org/10.1007/s11102-019-00944-0

Papleontiou-Louca, E. (2003). The concept and instruction of metacognition. *Teacher Development, 7*(1), 9–30.

Parvathaneni, A., & Das, J. (2021, June 30). *Balint Syndrome*. StatPearls. www.ncbi.nlm.nih.gov/books/NBK544347/

Patel, A., Biso, G., & Fowler, J. (2021, July 31). *Neuroanatomy, temporal lobe*. StatPearls. www.ncbi.nlm.nih.gov/books/NBK519512/

Rapoport, M., van Reekum, R., & Mayberg, H. (2000). The role of the cerebellum in cognition and behavior. *Journal of Neuropsychiatry and Clinical Neurosciences, 12*, 193–198. https://doi.org/10.1176/jnp.12.2.193

Rubin, R., Watson, P., Duff, M., & Cohen, N. (2014). The role of hippocampus in flexible cognition and social behavior. *Frontiers in Human Neuroscience, 8*, 1–12. https://doi.org/10.3389/fnhum.2014.00742

Sakai, J. (2020). Core Concept: How synaptic pruning shapes neural wiring during development and, possibly, in disease. *Proceedings of the National Academy of Sciences of the United States of America, 117*(28), 16096–16099. https://doi.org/10.1073/pnas.2010281117

Sargis, R. (2021, July 2). *An overview of the hypothalamus: The endocrine system's link to the nervous system*. EndocrineWeb. www.endocrineweb.com/endocrinology/overview-hypothalamus

Sav, A., Rotondo, F., Syro, L., Serna, C., & Kovacs, K. (2019). Pituitary pathology in traumatic brain injury: A review. *Pituitary, 22*(3), 201–211. https://doi.org/10.1007/s11102-019-00958-8

Seladi-Schulman, J. (2019, March 14). *The 12 cranial nerves*. Healthline. www.healthline.com/health/12-cranial-nerves

Shahid, Z., Asuka, E., & Singh, G. (2021, May 9). *Physiology, hypothalamus*. National Center for Biotechnology Information. www.ncbi.nlm.nih.gov/books/NBK535380/

Weber, M., Morrow, K., Rizer, W., Kangas, K., & Carlson, J. (2016). Sustained, not habituated, activity in the human amygdala: A pilot fMRI dot-probe study of attentional bias to fearful faces. *Cogent Psychology, 3*(1). https://doi.org/10.1080/23311908.2016.1259881

Westerhof-Evers, H., Fasotti, L., van der Naalt, J., & Spikman, J. (2019). Participation after traumatic brain injury: The surplus value of social cognition tests beyond measures for executive functioning and dysexecutive behavior in a statistical prediction model. *Brain Injury, 33*(1), 78–86.

Winslade, W. (1998). *Confronting traumatic brain injury: Devastation, hope, and healing*. Yale University Press.

Wright, A. (2020, October 10). *Limbic system: Amygdala*. Neuroscience Online. https://nba.uth.tmc.edu/neuroscience/m/s4/chapter06.html

Yang, Y., & Wang, J. (2017, October 31). *From structure to behavior in basolateral amygdala-hippocampus circuits*. Frontiers in Neural Circuits. https://doi.org/10.3389/fncir.2017.00086

6 Coping With Emotional and Social Deficits of Brain Injury

Case Study

Born into a pagan family, Ryan was assigned the role of family historian, which meant he was to memorize the family tree up to 300 generations. He grew up fascinated with history and eventually joined his country's military as a young adult. The military became his full-time career, where he flourished as a marksman and cultural expert. Ryan knew 12 languages and 47 dialects. He was riding in a tank when his company was blindsided by an enemy assault. Three of his comrades were killed, and Ryan was thrown from the tank and suffered multiple physical injuries and a traumatic brain injury. Given three days of rest, Ryan was sent back to his company and continued to serve until the end of his commission. Due to his injuries, he was unable to focus or shoot as accurately as before. He also struggled with sustained attention and concentration. Ryan developed a hair-trigger temper, which made it difficult for him to connect with his friends. His personality had changed from a serious, single-minded individual to a somewhat gregarious, emotionally volatile man. He took more risks and suffered another brain injury when he fell from a horse during a jousting tournament.

Ryan began dating an American who had been in his country on a mission trip. They fell in love, and Ryan asked for Lisa's hand in marriage. When Ryan became a Christian, his family disowned him. He moved to the United States and married Lisa. She did not know about his head injuries, much less how they affected his everyday life. Soon, she realized that Ryan had difficulty changing topics in conversation. He would talk incessantly about history, although he was unable to remember a list of groceries. His quick temper and short-term memory issues began to weigh on their relationship. Thankfully, Lisa was a mental health counselor who began studying about traumatic brain injury. She had conflicting feelings about Ryan. She loved him, but she was equally frustrated by his behavior, such as his inability to change course in a conversation, his inability to control his temper, his inability to participate in the give-and-take of a relationship, his poor social skills, and his inability to maintain friendships or keep a job. She became the sole breadwinner in the home and Ryan's full-time caregiver.

DOI: 10.4324/9781003301912-6

Through multiple trials, Ryan and Lisa came to workable coping strategies that eased the tension between them and prepared him for more meaningful friendships. For example, when Ryan would lose his temper, Lisa would leave him alone. After he calmed down, they were able to talk about what happened, such as what triggered the outburst and how they could manage it more effectively the next time. When Ryan would become verbose and perseverate on a topic, Lisa would gently squeeze his hand which was their agreed-upon signal that he needed to wrap up his thought and stop talking.

A frustration of Lisa's was the insensitivity of his friends and acquaintances, especially after she shared with them Ryan's challenges. It seemed they forgot because he "looked fine." Therefore, they expected him to be fine. Interestingly, Ryan found a kinship with members of the American Indian tribe near his home. They seemed to appreciate his knowledge and devotion to history, loyalty, and honesty. They taught Ryan how to create symbolic art, which he did with flair. Eventually, Ryan was able to modulate his verbal expression, practice give-and-take in conversation, and develop meaningful friendships. Lisa remains the breadwinner of the family.

An Invisible Injury

A key factor in the misunderstanding of brain injury is that people respond differently to visible injuries than they do to invisible disabilities (McClure, 2011). Although there is the risk of a stigma attached to visible disabilities, there is a disadvantage when a disability is invisible. A visible injury is often accommodated by others. For example, if one has a broken leg and is in a wheelchair, people tend to recognize, adjust, and go out of their way to assist. Also, people are unlikely to tell the injured person that his/her difficulty with walking is normal and will disappear in time, as many do when they address a person with a brain injury. Winslade (1998) stated that "only a fraction of the residual problems faced by brain-trauma victims are physical. The rest, the truly debilitating deficits, are mental and emotional." With brain injury, the severity is unseen and, often, unacknowledged. People tend to discount the complexity of the injury and suggest that the survivor will recover fully and return to his/her normal abilities. McClure (2011) pointed out that when people "have no markers of an injury that affects their behaviors, their appearance of normality and wellbeing leads people who do not understand brain injury to overlook any disability and fail to accommodate for it or offer appropriate rehabilitation." While there are social incentives to conceal a brain injury to avoid stigmatization, it can have damaging consequences when the brain injury is not recognized, which leads to unrealistic expectations, poor accommodations, and limited rehabilitation. In the counseling setting, the majority of brain injury survivors comment about how difficult it is when people do not acknowledge their injury because they look fine. Just as challenging is when family and friends who know about the injury do not accommodate it because the person looks the same as before the injury.

Overview of Emotional Deficits

Emotional deficits are one of the invisible sequelae of a traumatic brain injury. The ability to express and recognize emotions are skills fundamental to the human experience (Wearne et al., 2019). Emotions derive from one's personality and are built up from one's experience in one's environment. Growing up, one learns how to respond appropriately and to recognize fear, anger, sadness, and other emotions in one's body. The ability to control or direct one's own emotional expression is called emotional regulation (Kim et al., 2019). Difficulty with monitoring and inhibiting behavioral expressions of anger, irritability, or other negative emotions may result in behaviors that are contextually inappropriate (Verfaellie et al., 2012).

Brain injury alters the way one perceives the world and the way in which one controls one's reaction to it. Damage to the prefrontal cortex, brainstem, and limbic-related regions (i.e., hippocampus, amygdala) is linked to emotional dysregulation (Kim et al., 2019). In the early stages of brain injury recovery, there are two extremes of emotional expression (Gronwall et al., 1998). At one extreme, the individual may appear happy and unrealistically optimistic or elated, unaware or unconcerned about the effects of his/her brain injury. S/he may not express sadness when told information that should be distressing. At the other extreme, there is no emotion at all. As an example, one client came to the support group stating that he could not laugh or cry. He felt nothing. This gentleman knew enough to realize that this was not normal but was unable to find the "emotion button" that others appeared to have and that he had pre-injury. Another survivor of TBI stated that she could not cry even when she was sad. Unfortunately, one result of someone being unable to express emotion is that the individual may appear uncaring, unmoved, unloving, and uninterested.

Emotional disinhibition is another potential result of brain injury. Simply, the person with this sequela does not have a filter. S/he may say whatever comes to mind, whenever it comes to mind, not recognizing the inappropriateness of the comment. The lack of a filter will be discussed more thoroughly in the next chapter, which addresses cognitive deficits. However, it is important to recognize that disinhibition adversely affects social interactions and contributes to sensory overload. Not only does the person lack the ability to inhibit what s/he says, s/he also is not able to filter what comes in, such as environmental stimuli.

Emotional Lability

A brain injury causes the person to react differently to emotional situations. The brain-injured person may exhibit rapid mood swings, which means that s/he vacillates between high and low emotions. Brain injury mood swings and emotional lability are not the same thing as the mental illness mood swings of bipolar disorder. The emotional mood swings of brain injury can exhibit as frequent ups and downs, sometimes within the same conversation, whereas bipolar mood swings are characterized by periods of manic highs that can last for

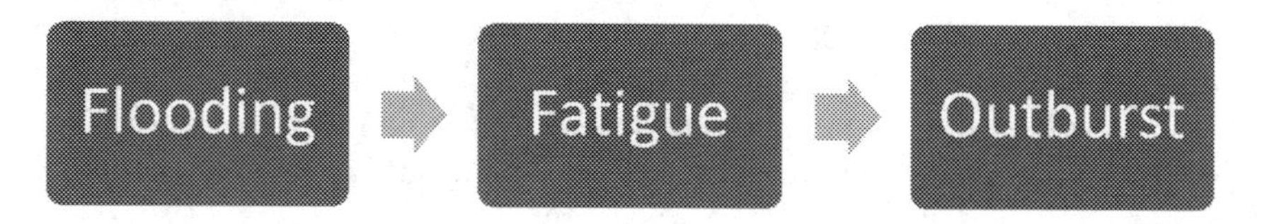

Figure 6.1 Progression to outbursts.

days to weeks and periods of depressive lows that can last the same amount of time. As one may imagine, emotional lability "may have deleterious effects on interpersonal relationships, reducing access to sources of social and economic support" (Verfaellie et al., 2012).

Additionally, the survivor may have difficulty controlling the expression of his/her emotions such as laughter or tears. Pseudobulbar affect (PBA) is the inability to control the outward expression of emotion, which is a disorder of the midbrain and is not to be confused with depression (Eames, 2001). Sometimes PBA manifests as the inability to regulate emotions long after the event stops or the experience of emotion for no reason at all. Other times, the person may cry when the situation calls for happiness or laugh when the situation is somber. Often it is a sudden, uncontrollable expression of crying or laughing minimally related to the situation. The good news is that emotional lability tends to stabilize as the brain recovers.

The control of emotional expression is often inhibited with fatigue. When a survivor of TBI is fatigued, s/he is less able to control his/her emotions. Irritability and aggression are outcomes of poor emotional control. For example, crowds of people, noise, and high sensory environments contribute to the individual feeling scared or confused, which can trigger an anger outburst. The environmental demands are sometimes referred to as "flooding" or sensory overload. The pattern noted in Figure 6.1 shows that sensory overload or flooding contributes to fatigue, which manifests as emotional outbursts.

Progression of Outbursts

Outbursts may include profanity, which many times was foreign to the individual pre-injury. It is important for the family to recognize the profanity as a part of the brain injury and not an indication of character. McClure (2011) stated that, when "caregivers attribute the behaviors to the person's personality, they experience more resentment and other negative effects." As paradoxical as it may seem, if a survivor has an emotional outburst, it is because s/he feels safe with the person and knows that s/he is loved. This feeling is not the same with friends, so the survivor spends a considerable amount of energy controlling his/her irritability, because s/he knows that if s/he "blows up" the person is likely to leave. Winslade (1998) described individuals with brain injury who have trouble controlling their anger and socially inappropriate impulses, but who can often do so with great effort in a structured environment. Therefore, when dealing with people outside of his/her family, the individual may appear normal for short periods of time. At home, the family becomes the "safety valve" and the survivor can let off steam (Gronwall et al., 1998). The verbal diatribes or abuse are especially painful when they are directed at a caregiver who has devoted him/herself to caring for the person who is lashing out (Winslade, 1998). However difficult, it is imperative for the family member to not take the outbursts personally, because the statements reflect organic damage, not personality. Comments that are impulsive, labile, acting out, apathetic, or disinterested stem from frontal lobe injury.

Social Deficits and Implications

Social cognition refers to the

> knowledge, processing, and application of culturally relevant (and often quite subtle) behaviour that assists in establishing and maintaining interpersonal relationships to varying degrees of intimacy and complexity – ranging from superficial "one-off" service encounters, through to grappling with the reactions of a partner during an emotionally charged argument.
>
> (Snow, 2013)

It incorporates one's ability to understand, predict, and interpret the beliefs and feelings of others. It also involves the ability to practice social inferencing. According to Snow (2013), social inferencing "refers to the ability to derive intended meaning from incomplete or contradictory verbal/non-verbal information that is shared in a particular social context." Wood (2001) explained that the neurobehavioral disability comprising attention deficits, diminished insight, poor social judgment, lability, problems with impulse control, and personality changes leads to a serious social handicap. Adaptive social behavior involves the ability to simultaneously process incoming information, monitor one's response, evaluate its social impact, and decide whether the response is appropriate or needs to be changed (Wood, 2001). Unfortunately, brain injury survivors may have an inability to use their intelligence "in a meaningful and socially adaptive way, such as to monitor, inhibit, or alter behaviours, which others find offensive, threatening, or embarrassing" (Wood, 2001). The inability to regulate emotional behavior contributes to social dysfunction (Kim et al., 2019). The ever-changing processing of information in often noisy social environments contributes to social maladjustment. Often, brain injury survivors need to relearn social graces and appropriate social behaviors, such as politeness, turn-taking in conversation, nonverbal cues, and use of cooperative gestures such as waving one's hand to say hello or goodbye. When the individual does not behave appropriately, especially in public, it is a source of embarrassment to the family and caregivers. Additionally, onlookers are unaware of how to manage such behaviors in a respectful manner, thereby magnifying the problem.

In their study from the University of New South Wales, Australia, Wearne et al. (2019) explained that emotional expression communicates feelings, attitudes, and the intent of the expresser. It also entails the ability to quickly assess and process cues of situational context. Therefore, emotional expression "represents an important factor underlying the understanding of social contexts requisite for social and interpersonal relationships." The ability to express emotion appropriately is crucial to nonverbal communication and is associated with successful interpersonal functioning and the effective demonstration of social skills (Wearne et al., 2019). The researchers also found that explicit, subjective experience of emotion is key in recognizing the emotional displays of others, "including facial mimicry, the sharing of subjective emotional states, and body representations and/or postures." Simply put, survivors of TBI may have difficulty experiencing or assigning meaning to emotions (alexithymia). They may also have problems interpreting emotional meaning through auditory channels, such tone of voice, rate of speech, volume, or intonational contour (Snow, 2013).

The reduction in social support and activities contributes to a lower quality of life (Kelly et al., 2013). Immediately after the injury, family and friends come to their loved one's aid. They provide support and hope and prayers that the brain injury survivor will return to his/her "old self." As the days, weeks, and months pass, visits decline and people move on with their own lives. As the survivor recovers, his/her emotional deficits become more obvious. S/he often is unable to identify emotional reactions from others due to damage to the connecting pathways between the amygdala and the temporal lobe. This deficit in awareness of others manifests as difficulty recognizing whether the other person is sad or happy by his/her facial expressions. This leads to an uncomfortable and awkward social interaction. Unfortunately, instead of trying to communicate and correct the miscue, most individuals separate themselves from the survivor. Undesirable behaviors are unfairly attributed to the survivor's personality rather than to the brain injury (McClure, 2011).

Hoofien et al. (2001) found that the primary concern for family members was the person's personality change, but the primary concern for survivors was the lack of social contacts. One of the most debilitating consequences of a severe traumatic brain injury is the loss of social contacts and social functioning (Long et al., 2008). Because of the inability to maintain friendships or create new friends, survivors rely disproportionately upon parents and spouses for emotional support (Ponsford et al., 1995). Increased social activity "is associated with both lower levels of depression and higher levels of positive affect" (Brown et al., 2003). However, with the difficulty of generating emotional expression befitting the circumstances, social acceptance is limited or nonexistent. This is one of the main reasons that Hope After Brain Injury hosts a movie and dinner evening once a quarter. A local theatre is rented for brain injury survivors and their families to practice healthy social activities within a safe environment. The participants are given an opportunity to order their meal, choose the movie, and create new friendships with others who have experienced similar injuries.

Coping With Emotional and Social Deficits

Education is the first line of defense in coping with emotional and social deficits. Knowledge of how brain injury can adversely affect one's emotions and behaviors helps the family members and caregivers understand that these are organic issues, not personality issues. The second line of defense is to identify external factors. A quick assessment of environmental stimuli and modification if needed will help to alleviate sensory overload. Consider the various external influences such as noise level, brightness, number and proximity of people, landscaping sounds, room temperature, and time pressure. Is the radio on? Is the television loud? Are there more than a couple of people in the same room? Is there cross-talk? Are the lights too bright? Is the climate in the room too cold or too hot? Is there time pressure? Often people with brain injury are unable to filter the external stimulation, so that they are often overwhelmed. Ensuring a quiet space to which they can retreat will help to manage the flooding experience. Elimination of the trigger events and circumstances will go a long way toward managing emotions and improving social interactions.

The following are some practical suggestions for the loved one who has the brain injury to implement when confronted with conflictual experiences. Some of these are contingent on the phase of recovery.

1. Walk. Physical exercise helps work out emotional overload.
2. Create a safe, quiet space to retreat to when emotionally or environmentally overwhelmed.
3. Journal. Writing in a journal has two purposes. One is expression and the other is exploration. It is helpful to express what one feels in the non-judgmental zone of a journal. Additionally, in the writing itself, sometimes one may discover what contributes to the actual irritation or frustration. For example, someone may have said something that triggered a feeling of insecurity or vulnerability or abandonment.
4. Inform one's family and friends that comments are not to be taken personally.
5. Apologize when one's comments are hurtful or abusive.
6. Practice stopping, breathing, and separating when overwhelmed. Deep breathing is a common technique one can use to help calm down.
7. Avoid triggers.
8. Create a signal with a family member that can be used at the beginning of an outburst.
9. Rest. Managing fatigue is essential for constructive emotional expression and meaningful social interaction.
10. Create a flexible routine. Flexibility alleviates the constant readjusting required for changing plans but offers the space to accommodate a new opportunity.
11. Practice listening without interrupting.
12. Communicate gratitude.

13 Consider joining a support group of other brain injury survivors. Hearing from others about their experiences can help one not feel alone or different. A healthy support group offers a safe space to practice social interactions while making friends who understand.

The following are suggestions for caregivers and family members to consider while working with a loved one with a brain injury. Again, some of these are contingent on his/her ability to respond, depending on the phase of recovery.

1. Celebrate the small successes. Remember that the brain injury survivor is learning to live again. The small things are huge to him/her. For example, congratulate a survivor for relearning to brush his/her teeth, which requires concentration and the use of fine motor skills.
2. Encourage. Staying positive goes a long way in creating an encouraging and hope-filled environment.
3. Trust the process. Although slow, brain injury recovery comes in small steps over incremental pieces of time. Neuroplasticity is in play but is not immediately evident.
4. Interpret emotional outbursts as signals instead of insults. Most of the time, an emotional outburst is related to flooding and fatigue. Although harsh, it is not meant to offend. Taking the comments personally sets up an unnecessary argument. Being critical and holding grudges, however justified, do little to remedy a disagreement.
5. Debrief. After an outburst, the survivor is often apologetic. At this point, it is good to discuss what happened and help him/her come up with a different, more effective way of expressing frustration or anger.
6. Create a sign that signals a break is needed. Encourage the loved one to separate and calm down.
7. Employ one's own support system. Educate friends and family about the brain injury. Ask them to be a listening, nonjudgmental resource.
8. Exercise. Getting away alone to physically work out frustrations is healthy.
9. Take vitamins. One's health as the caregiver needs to be primary.
10. Breathe and practice meditation or other spiritual observations; say mantras or prayers. This helps to calm the spirit and center oneself.
11. Journal. As mentioned earlier, writing holds space for expression and exploration of feelings and experiences. It also holds a timeline of recovery that can be helpful and hopeful during different phases of recovery.
12. Allow friends to help with errands and appointments.
13. Create flexible routines. Knowing what to expect in the day goes a long way toward avoiding undue stress that can accompany a loose schedule.
14. Consider joining a support group for caregivers of individuals with brain injury. Resources and understanding are among the greatest needs for caregivers. In a healthy support group, these needs are met along with the development of comradery and friendships with people who understand the challenges of brain injury.

15 Practice patience. The brain injury road is long and arduous. It is consistently inconsistent, which is good to remember because sometimes happy, rewarding moments can be interspersed amid challenging moments. Being patient with oneself and others is a needed, life-giving gift.

These suggestions for the survivor and caregiver offer techniques, space, and time to navigate one of the most challenging terrains of recovery.

Conclusion

The emotional and social deficits that accompany brain injury were discussed in this chapter. Emotional deficits are one of the "invisible" aspects of brain injury. Emotional lability and the expression of no emotion were addressed, along with recognition of the pseudobulbar affect common to severe traumatic brain injury. The recognition that these deficits are organic in nature and not a reflection of personality or character is essential to not taking the emotional and social disinhibitions personally. The social awkwardness and need for social intelligence were also addressed. It is worth noting that the emotional outbursts and social inappropriateness do improve over time with proper instruction and encouragement. The progression of outbursts from sensory overload and fatigue originates from my practice and experience with brain injury survivors and their families. Suggestions for survivors and their families were outlined as stepping-stones to their mental and emotional health. The next chapter will discuss the cognitive deficits associated with brain injury and how these issues contribute to such issues as lack of self-awareness, memory loss, egocentricity, communication issues, poor judgment, decreased attention, and disinhibition.

References

Brown, M., Gordon, W., & Spielman, L. (2003). Participation in social and recreational activity in the community by individuals with traumatic brain injury. *Rehabilitation Psychology*, *48*(4), 266–274. https://doi.org/10.1037/0090-5550.48.4.266

Eames, P. (2001). Distinguishing the neuropsychiatric, psychiatric, and psychological consequences of acquired brain injury. In R. Wood & T. McMillan (Eds.), *Neurobehavioural disability and social handicap following traumatic brain injury* (pp. 29–45). Psychology Press.

Gronwall, D., Wrightson, P., & Waddell, P. (1998). *Head injury: The facts* (2nd ed.). Oxford University Press.

Hoofien, D., Gilboa, A., Vakil, E., & Donovick, P. (2001). Traumatic brain injury (TBI) 10–20 years later: A comprehensive outcome study of psychiatric symptomology, cognitive abilities and psychosocial functioning. *Brain Injury*, *15*(3), 189–209.

Kelly, M., McDonald, S., & Kellet, D. (2013). The psychological effects of ostracism following traumatic brain injury. *Brain Injury*, *27*(13–14), 1676–1684. https://doi.org/10.3109/02699052.2013.834381

Kim, S., Zemon, V., Lehrer, P., McCraty, R., Cavallo, M., Raghavan, P., Ginsberg, J., & Foley, F. (2019). Emotion regulation after acquired brain injury: A study of heart rate variability, attentional control, and psychophysiology. *Brain Injury*, *33*(8), 1012–1020. https://doi.org/10.1080/02699052.2019.1593506

Long, E., McDonald, S., Tate, R., Togher, L., & Bornhofen, C. (2008). Assessing social skills in people with very severe traumatic brain injury: Validity of the Social Performance Survey Schedule (SPSS). *Brain Impairment*, *9*(3), 274–281.

McClure, J. (2011). The role of causal attributions in public misconceptions about brain injury. *Rehabilitation Psychology*, *56*(2), 85–93.

Ponsford, J., Olver, J., & Curran, C. (1995). A profile of outcome: 2 years after traumatic brain injury. *Brain Injury*, *9*(1), 1–10. https://doi.org/10.3109/02699059509004565

Snow, P. (2013). Communication competence following TBI. In J. Ponsford, S. Sloan, & P. Snow (Eds.), *Traumatic brain injury: Rehabilitation for everyday adaptive living* (2nd ed., pp. 133–163). Psychology Press.

Verfaellie, M., Amick, M., & Vasterling, J. (2012). Effects of traumatic brain injury – Associated neurocognitive alterations on posttraumatic stress disorder. In J. Vasterling, R. Bryant, & T. Keane (Eds.), *PTSD and mild traumatic brain injury* (pp. 82–102). The Guilford Press.

Wearne, T., Osborne-Crowley, K., Rosenberg, H., Dethier, M., & McDonald, S. (2019). Emotion recognition depends on subjective emotional experience and not on facial expressivity: Evidence from traumatic brain injury. *Brain Injury*, *33*(1), 12–22. https://doi.org/10.1080/02699052.2018.1531300

Winslade, W. (1998). *Confronting traumatic brain injury: Devastation, hope, and healing*. Yale University Press.

Wood, R. (2001). Understanding neurobehavioural disability. In R. Wood & T. MacMillan (Eds.), *Neurobehavioural disability and social handicap following traumatic brain injury* (pp. 1–28). Psychology Press.

7 Coping With Cognitive Deficits of Brain Injury

Case Study

Susan, 61, was 13 months away from celebrating her silver anniversary as an executive with a global investment banking company. Unfortunately, a series of falls abruptly ended her career. After her third fall in as many months, Susan could no longer manage the drive to her job or navigate the complexity of her position as a risk management specialist. Prior to her accidents, Susan was detail-oriented, shrewd, funny, politically savvy, highly intelligent, and well respected. She could break down complicated concepts for her subordinates or communicate in the language of an investor. It was common for Susan to create step-by-step instructions detailing specific job responsibilities or procedures should someone need assistance. After her falls, Susan could not follow those same instructions. She suffered three mild traumatic brain injuries that adversely affected her ability to comprehend, process, or speak fluently. She experienced double vision and tinnitus and was unable see three dimensionally. Initially, her physicians did not recognize the severity of her brain injuries because she could not report a loss of consciousness. They recommended rest and return to work in a week. Not long into her day after she returned to work, she found herself confused and unable to comprehend a conversation. She would miss meetings that she scheduled and, if she did remember, she was unable to lead the meeting. She struggled with dizziness, sensory overload, aphasia, balance issues, inability to recognize time, and slowed reflexes. When she stood up to walk, she had to hold onto the wall to keep from falling. She stated that it was a miracle that she drove on the highway without causing a wreck.

After some days of trying to work, Susan returned to her physician who referred her to a neurologist. The neurologist promptly took her out of work and placed her on disability. Susan began a series of therapies including physical, occupational, and speech therapy. After being approved for long-term disability, the company eventually recommended that Susan take early retirement, which she did. Susan regretted the decision, even though she knew it was the right choice and a generous gesture from her company. With speech therapy, Susan was eventually able to find the right words in a conversation and speak fluently. Her aphasia only returns when she is fatigued.

DOI: 10.4324/9781003301912-7

The cognitive exercises in her therapy sessions were extremely challenging for Susan. One hour of therapy would cost her two days in bed. Previously an expert in multitasking and higher-level thinking, Susan struggled to complete simple tasks. It took her an extended amount of time to figure out how to solve a simple math problem. As mentioned, pre-injury Susan was highly intelligent, organized, well-spoken, humorous, straightforward, and kind. Since her injuries, she has slower processing and difficulty with awareness, and she is irritable and ultrasensitive to light and sounds. She fears that her IQ has diminished and that her ability to think has decreased. The therapy regimen helped her to develop cognitive strategies to improve her memory and compensatory skills to accommodate deficiencies.

Eventually, Susan graduated from her physical, occupational, and speech therapies. She continues to work with a vestibular therapist, who helps with her residual balance and vision issues. She has learned to minimize sensory overload and maximize task accomplishment by utilizing her cognitive skills during times when she feels fresh and energetic. She and her husband have moved into a smaller, one-story house that has no stairs. Susan is acclimating to a slower lifestyle. She still grieves the premature ending of her successful career. Currently, she is trying to learn to cook again and to take care of household chores. Her children and grandchildren visit often, which brings her joy.

Cognition Defined

Cognition is the act of thinking or knowing. When someone experiences a traumatic or acquired brain injury, cognitive processes are affected. Executive function, first coined by Muriel Lezak in 1982, is the mental capacity to engage successfully in independent, purposive, self-serving behavior. Executive function, a major function of the frontal lobe, is divided into four components: formulation of goals, planning, development, and execution (Lezak, 1982). Some of the functions affected are attention and concentration, processing and understanding information, memory, planning and organizing, reasoning, problem-solving, self-awareness, judgment, and social behavior. Cognitive rehabilitation (the process of restoring cognitive function) is then crucial for the recovery process (Stratton & Gregory, 1994).

Attention and Concentration Deficits

Attention as described by Tsaousides and Gordon (2009) is a "complex mental activity that refers to how an individual receives and begins to process internal and external stimuli." People with brain injury have difficulty paying attention and/or staying focused. Attention problems and a reduced capacity to process information are among the most frequently reported problems after brain injury (Himanen et al., 2009). Survivors complain of slowed thinking, difficulty concentrating, increased distractibility and inability to return to a task once distracted, and difficulty attending to more than one thing at a time.

They also complain that cognitive functioning is more effortful and can cause headaches, fatigue, and irritability (Cicerone, 1996). Poor attention is "a disruption of functions mediated by the frontal and medial temporal regions of the brain" (Verfaellie et al., 2012). Every waking moment one must allocate the appropriate attentional resources to plan activities, respond to unexpected events, select appropriate behavioral responses, and evaluate the success of one's performance to guide future behavior. Studies have found that the frontal cortex, parietal cortex, thalamic, and brainstem regions support attention-related behavior (Eckert et al., 2009). Attention has been subdivided into "systems that support executive function (problem solving or goal-directed behavior), selection or direction of attention, and arousal" (Eckert et al., 2009). The deficits of brain injury affect alertness/arousal, selective attention, and "energetic aspects of attention, which include such components as effort, resource allocation, and speed of processing" (Niemann et al., 1996). Although individuals with depression may exhibit cognitive slowness, according to a study from Turku University Central Hospital between 1966–1972, attention functions are independent of depressive symptoms and "depression should not be considered as a causative factor in all the cognitive deficits in chronic TBI" (Himanen et al., 2009).

Gronwall et al. (1998) address attention and concentration from three perspectives. Focused attention is concentration on one thing. A brain-injured individual finds it difficult not to be distracted by trivial noises or movements. The mechanism that helps one keep track of a select item is damaged. Second, divided attention between two or more things at the same time is difficult for a survivor of TBI. If s/he cannot focus on one task, it is unlikely s/he will be able to focus on two. The third way that this cognitive deficit manifests is in a poor attention span. The person has the inability to concentrate on a task for an extended period. In the early stages of recovery, the attention span is quite short. As the person improves, his/her ability to maintain focused attention increases, although the length of time is dependent on fatigue level.

Managing Attention and Concentration Deficits

A survivor with TBI who struggles with attention and concentration will require assistance to incorporate several coping strategies. The first suggestion is to eliminate as many distractions as possible. This may mean secluding the individual to help him/her focus. Remember that fatigue decreases the ability to focus. An attempt to accomplish a cognitive task will be more successful when the survivor is well rested. Additionally, one should not talk to an individual while s/he is trying to concentrate. For example, if a survivor of TBI is walking and trying to focus on his/her balance and gait, speaking to him/her at the same time is not helpful.

The division of tasks into small, achievable parts is especially important when someone is unable to concentrate. One client stated that she can only do "onesies," meaning she can only do a task that requires one step, such as brushing her hair. The removal of distractions such as nonessentials from countertops or living spaces can help decrease distractibility and improve attention. In a social atmosphere, position the survivor away from the crowd so that his/her attention can be limited to who is in the direct line of vision.

Because fatigue decreases one's ability to concentrate, it may be helpful to plan to do more complicated tasks in the morning or when the person feels fresh and alert. It is also recommended that, when the brain injury survivor gets tired, it is better that s/he rests rather than pushing through to complete the task. To try to finish a goal in one setting when fatigued will most likely result in a failed effort. Interestingly, when a survivor of TBI is fatigued, s/he is less likely to want to rest and will try to push through. Another factor contributing to the successful completion of tasks is the removal of any time limit. The pressure of trying to accomplish something in a set amount of time increases fatigue and irritability and decreases the ability to attend and concentrate.

Some researchers have recognized the role of computer-assisted training as a useful tool to improve general cognitive processing. They have shown that computer-assisted strategies may "improve attention, memory, and executive skills" (Barman et al., 2016). Other uses for this mode of assistance extend to memory training, attention, problem-solving, and job assimilation (Tsaousides & Gordon, 2009). Various researchers have studied the validity of these programs with mixed results. While the survivor may perform well on computerized games, the skills may not be readily transferrable to real-life situations.

Processing and Understanding Deficits

After a brain injury, the survivor's information processing often slows down and is more challenging. This is reflected in his/her difficulty understanding what others are saying. S/he may require more time to process and follow instructions. Comprehension of a plot on television or in a movie is impaired, as is attention to a program with a lot of movement such as sports. More time is needed to read and understand written information, such as closed captioning, books, magazines, or social media.

Another aspect of processing and understanding is problem-solving. Deficits in this area can be a significant obstacle to successful community reintegration because they prevent individuals with TBI from returning to productive personal and vocational lives. Problem-solving has been defined as "a goal-directed cognitive activity that arises in situations from which there is no immediately apparent or available response" (Rath et al., 2003). Deficits in problem-solving have been characterized as deficiencies in purposeful, logical, and analytical thought due to brain damage (von Cramon & Matthes-von Cramon, 1992). An extension of problem-solving is social problem-solving, which refers to "problem solving as it occurs in everyday life; the adjective *social* does not restrict problem solving to any particular domain but instead indicates that problem solving occurs in the everyday social environment" (Rath et al., 2003).

An important aspect of slowed processing is the inability to recognize warning signs in a timely fashion. Therefore, it is imperative to limit or avoid driving or other high-risk activities. The slowness also pertains to daily tasks such as getting ready for the day. According to Cicerone (1996), decreased processing speed appears "to be a primary factor in limiting attention." He also noted that deficits of processing speed are not reflective of accuracy. Meaning, the speed at which the individual processes the information does not adversely affect the correct outcome.

Problem-solving and making decisions are also difficult. When processing is impaired, the survivor is inflexible, cannot consider various solutions, or acts too quickly without recognizing the repercussions of the action. An example of everyday problem-solving is generating a solution that adheres to time and resource restraints. Another difficulty is when the individual cannot predict when problems may arise and therefore is not prepared with alternatives when they are needed. Still other survivors are unable to organize and prioritize steps to solve a problem (Kennedy et al., 2008). One of the survivors stated that she wished she had a picture of an hourglass to let people know that she is thinking, but is as slow as an hourglass.

Managing Processing and Understanding Deficits

Remembering to slow down when one is communicating with a survivor of TBI is key to increasing his/her ability to process and understand. Give small amounts of information at a time and pause occasionally for processing to set up a successful interaction. Stopping one's internal clock when working with survivors will help the speaker to slow down and allow him/her to better understand exactly what is being said. Inherent in caregiving is constantly thinking of and anticipating the next thing, which inadvertently puts pressure on the loved one. Slower is better. As the loved one improves, the pace of communication can be increased. Be willing to repeat yourself, and ask the survivor to repeat what s/he heard to ensure understanding. Encourage note-taking and utilization of his/her diary or organizer to summarize. When watching television with a survivor of TBI, consider a show with limited movement and a singular message, such as animation, or a show with limited or simple story lines.

Sometimes it is helpful to have a family member help to walk the individual through a problem-solving process. For example, name the problem and possible solutions within the time frame and resources allotted. Second, list the pros and cons of each possible solution. Third, choose a solution and try it. Finally, evaluate the outcome of the solution. As the survivor learns to navigate his/her world, it is recommended that s/he choose a family member or two whom s/he trusts and with whom s/he can discuss various life decisions. Help the survivor to solve a problem rather than solving the problem for him/her. Give him/her extra time to consider the issue and possible solutions. This may involve offering alternative solutions and outcomes as a means of exploration and concluding appropriately. Keep in mind that the individual's processing is slower, and note that it make take more time to resolve an issue.

Cognitive Rehabilitation Therapy

Cognitive rehabilitation therapy (CRT) refers to "a wide group of activities and techniques designed to retrain higher brain functions and compensate for deficits with newly-acquired strategies" (Saux et al., 2014). The goal is "to improve the person's ability to perform cognitive tasks, cope with affective [emotional] distress, and increase self-confidence, self-efficacy, and self-awareness" (Tsaousides & Gordon, 2009). Although there are a variety of techniques, basically there are two approaches to CRT. One is restorative and the other is compensatory. The restorative approach includes retraining previously learned skills and using residual abilities. The compensatory approach teaches ways of bypassing or compensating for the impaired function, which includes making environmental adjustments and accommodating the cognitive impairments to increase self-awareness and acceptance (Barman et al., 2016). According to Tsaousides and Gordon (2009), CRT is applicable at all stages of recovery, in different settings, with different modalities such as individual, family, and couples counseling, and by professionals from different disciplines such as speech-language pathologists, occupational therapists, and neuropsychologists.

CRT for attention deficits may include flashcards to improve basic attention skills. Attention Process Training (APT) was developed by Sohlberg and Mateer (1987) and incorporates practicing processes to improve visual and auditory attention. For example, a patient is asked to listen to an audio track and to press a button when a certain word is said. Competence is achieved when the individual successfully masters a skill level and graduates to a higher skill level.

CRT for memory deficits includes techniques "such as face-name associations, memory for past events, prospective memory, and learning new information" (Tsaousides & Gordon, 2009). The restorative exercises include word list memorization, visual imagery, paragraph recall, and use of mnemonics. Compensatory strategies for memory include memory notebooks, technology helps such as lists on one's cell phone or software applications, voice recorders, and sticky notes that can be attached to one's computer or desk. One client stated that his phone is his "second brain." Memory notebooks may have sections such as a calendar, appointment lists, to-do lists, address and contact lists, and names of providers. A young survivor of ABI stated she kept a log of her emotions on each page. She also wrote a list of her accomplishments each day. Another survivor of a brain aneurysm kept a log of what the barometric pressure was each given day. He believed that his brain fog was directly associated with the atmospheric pressure. In this case, his list was both compensatory and informative.

Metacognition is the "ability to think about thinking and occurs with self-regulation" (Copley et al., 2015). Its two main functions are to monitor one's thoughts and to then use that information to alter and improve one's thinking and behavior. Metacognition strategy instruction (MSI) is a CRT approach that helps individuals to gain awareness by self-monitoring, identifying and correcting errors, and generating strategies for future tasks. The four specific steps to MSI are (1) set a goal, (2) compare current performance with goals, (3) decide how to alter behavior to meet goals, and (4) implement new behavior (Kennedy et al., 2008). Copley et al. (2015) added a fifth step which was to self-predict future behavior or strategies as this builds awareness and application to real environment experiences. MSI is a recommended strategy for adults with TBI who struggle with problem-solving, planning, and organization (Kennedy et al., 2008).

Memory Deficits

Memory loss is one of the most common complaints of brain injury survivors, with a prevalence ranging from 54% to 84% (Chiaravalloti et al., 2015). Memory includes difficulty encoding new information and recalling past events. Such deficits have an adverse effect on multiple aspects of everyday life, such as occupational, emotional, and social functioning and activities of daily living. Metamemory is defined as "one's knowledge, awareness, and beliefs about the functioning of one's own memory" (Kit et al., 2007). According to Bandura (1989), the degree to which an individual seeks out a memory-demanding situation, puts an effort into memory tasks, and has expectations surrounding memory performance is determined, at least in part, by metamemory. Sometimes a person will remember parts of a story or event but not the whole thing. When this happens, the survivor's brain will try to fill in the blank and comes up with a false memory. This is called confabulation. It is important to remember that confabulation is a way to make sense of an event for the survivor. Even though the memory is false, it is not meant to be a lie. The intent is to make sense, not to mislead or deceive. Many times, the person does not recognize that the information is fabricated.

Managing Memory Deficits

Improving memory functioning is paramount to improving quality of life. Organization and structure are mainstays of memory improvement. Internal aids such as visual imagery are more effective for memory issues within the mild traumatic brain injury population. However, there is strong evidence surrounding the effectiveness of external aids as compensatory strategies for daily memory problems (Rees et al., 2007). An example of an external aid is to place commonly used items in the same location. Mail, important papers, and other items are assigned their own places in the house. A white board or calendar in a common area that lists appointments and tasks for the week can reduce memory mishaps. Setting an alarm on a cell phone or other device can signal the time to take medication. A structured routine includes set times to wake up, eat, and retire for the evening. This may also include choosing times to complete certain activities of daily living, such as laundry, exercise, rest, and participation in family events. The creation of a to-do list with the most important task listed at the top helps the writer know in what order to complete the tasks. Other external aids include a memory notebook dedicated to specific organizational needs and an appointment planner is that lists times and dates of appointments per week, per month, and per year.

Improving memory requires the individual to devote time to learn new activities and practice new information. Linking new information to a previous experience can be helpful in learning a new activity. Writing down step-by-step instructions is helpful both cognitively and physically to create a new memory. Recording conversations can also help in keeping up with new information. Smaller steps help to develop the feeling of accomplishment and mastery. Encouraging individuals to focus more on memory successes rather than failures contributes to a better sense of identity (Kit et al., 2007).

Lack of Awareness

According to Crosson et al. (1989), awareness is the ability to recognize problems caused by impaired brain function. If a survivor has a lack of awareness, also called anosognosia, s/he may not be able to recognize his/her need for rehabilitation and may prematurely terminate participation in treatment, thereby reducing his/her opportunity and capacity to adopt compensatory strategies (Richardson et al., 2014). Awareness deficits have been associated with "poorer long-term rehabilitation, vocational and social outcomes" (Malouf et al., 2014). Studies have also found that individuals who are more aware of their deficits show better treatment performance and have better rehabilitation outcomes, including successful work re-entry (Wallace & Bogner, 2000). Interestingly, studies have found that participants who reported fewer deficits also experienced less depression and anxiety (Wallace & Bogner, 2000).

Fleming and Strong (1995) divided lack of awareness into three categories: (1) awareness of the impairments caused by the brain injury, (2) awareness of the functional implications of the injury such as driving, work, etc., and (3) awareness conceived as the ability to set realistic goals. Of the cognitive deficits, "the most difficult of these are the flawed judgment and inability to understand and acknowledge [a survivor's] remaining limitations" (Winslade, 1998). Muriel Lezak (1988) stated that,

> [B]y and large, as the severity of the organic damage increases, the capacity for self-awareness, and particularly for accurate self-appreciation, decreases. Thus, the most profoundly impaired patients . . . are typically only dimly aware of their dysfunctions, if at all.

Work by Gasquoine (1992) found that there was a distinction between recognizing that there was an impairment and understanding the severity of the impairment. Generally, survivors of TBI "have been found to under-report their limitations in non-physical areas of functioning (i.e., cognitive and emotional functioning), while showing relatively better awareness of their limitations in physical areas of functioning (i.e. physical and sensory functioning)" (Malouf et al., 2014). The physical deficits are more concrete and recognizable and therefore less open to interpretation. The self-ratings of survivors about their functioning are typically higher than the ratings of family members and clinicians, including neuropsychological testing (Allen & Ruff, 1990). Malouf et al. (2014) study found that families rated survivors as having more severe functional impairments than did clinicians. Sometimes the lack of awareness may be due to poor executive function and reduced abstract reasoning, making it difficult for the person to connect poor performance to cognitive deficits (Dirette, 2002).

Another distinction in awareness is the survivor's awareness of future function versus current function. Future functions include driving a vehicle or maintaining a job. Survivors "have more difficulty appreciating how their impairments will affect their ability when they need to project themselves into the future to understand the difference between what they hope to happen and what will actually occur because of their impairments" (Malouf et al., 2014). This lack of insight causes problems when it comes to operating a motor vehicle. One client fell from a ladder at work and suffered a severe traumatic brain injury. He was unaware of the deficits caused by the injury, which created significant conflict between him and his wife. His workplace recommended that he retire, but he was set on returning to work stating that he was fine and did not have any deficits. The lack of awareness also contributed to him being unable to fully appreciate therapy or treatment recommendations because "everything was fine."

Managing Lack of Awareness

According to Dirette (2002), compensatory strategies are "techniques used by an individual with ABI to circumvent a deficit caused by impaired brain function." One of the strategies utilized in Dirette's study was pacing, which is "slowing down the input of information to decrease proactive interference and increase information processing." A frequent recommendation that I make to my patients is to "add grace to your pace," meaning do not rush ahead or put pressure on oneself to perform when it is not necessary. Slowing the speed of an interaction offers space to perceive, process, and understand information. It also eliminates or at least decreases mistakes, frustrations, and misperceptions. In counseling with the client mentioned in the previous paragraph, it was helpful to invite his wife to the sessions to address areas of improvement, such as communication. In this case, the incorporation of external help such as home health attendants assisted the client in recognizing that he could benefit from their oversight with medication, balance, transportation, and other activities of daily living. Eventually, he was able to accept their help and appreciate their efforts to keep him safe.

One of the difficulties for survivors of TBI is their comparison of present function versus pre-injury function. If a survivor has the memory to recall his/her previous level of function, s/he tends to compare his/her present self with that past self. The participants in Dirette's study (2002) found that "comparing their current performance to their premorbid performance was critical in developing awareness of cognitive deficits." The other significant finding was that participating in functional activities helped the participants gain awareness of their ability. So, it is important to create "real-life" situations and settings to develop awareness (Dirette, 2002).

Several authors caution the use of functional activities to improve awareness of deficits, because some clients may have an adverse psychological experience associated with gaining awareness of their deficits. It may be more helpful for the survivor to participate in a structured cognitive rehabilitation program after s/he has spent time at home. The increased awareness gained in a supervised setting can offer the psychological support needed to navigate any adverse reactions (Dirette, 2002). As an individual begins to perceive changes within him/herself associated with the brain injury, the adjustment becomes more challenging emotionally. The increase in emotional distress for the survivor and his/her family members contributes to depression and anxiety (this will be addressed in subsequent chapters). One of the recommendations is to encourage the survivor and his/her caregiver to do their best to not compare the person with the TBI to the person without the TBI. Although natural, it is an unfair comparison. To appropriately manage the emotional distress accompanying awareness is to practice a fair comparison. What is the survivor's current function as opposed to his/her function immediately following the injury? Recognizing the progress instead of seeing only deficits contributes to a more positive outlook.

Self-awareness does tend to improve over time. As noted, the awareness of physical changes typically precedes that of the cognitive and behavioral changes. Richardson et al. (2014) investigated the trajectory of self-awareness within the first year after a TBI and the concurrent biopsychosocial factors. They found that females showed a higher level of accurate goal-setting than males, although at one year post-injury, both genders were consistent with their goal-setting abilities, which may indicate that women are more likely to readily acknowledge their current difficulties that may impact future plans. Regarding the timing of increased awareness, their study suggested that compensatory strategies be introduced 6–12 months post-injury as awareness was better in that time frame.

Disinhibition

Frontal lobe damage may produce disinhibition in the survivor. Disinhibition is defined as a series of characteristics such as coarse behavior, overfamiliarity, inappropriate sexual behavior, gross errors of judgment, tactlessness, a marked indifference to the effects of one's actions on another person, and a lack of concern for the future consequences of one's behavior (Stratton & Gregory, 1994). Other behaviors of disinhibition include saying the first thing that springs to mind without recognition of the social appropriateness, breaking confidences, divulging too much personal information, and being unable to hide or contain emotions such as overreacting or acting aggressively toward another person. Basically, disinhibition interferes with the person's "ability to inhibit automatic behaviors, urges, and emotions and impedes goal-directed behavior, such as resisting temptation, delaying gratification, and controlling impulses" (Knutson et al., 2015). Ponsford (2013) stated that people with a TBI are, by virtue of their disability, sexually frustrated. Because of their reduced behavioral control, this may be expressed inappropriately such as crude talk or sexual advances.

Managing Disinhibition

There are different ways to manage disinhibition or inappropriate social behavior. Ponsford (2013) suggested educating the family and their brain-injured loved one that the behavior is a result of frontal lobe damage and that, with time and coping strategies, the behavior can be managed. It is important to remind them that there is the possibility that their loved one may say or do something without thinking and out of character. If possible, they should ignore the behavior and address the issue in private. Moving on to another topic of conversation or distracting the survivor is helpful. Respond to appropriate behavior with attention and praise. Inappropriate social behavior is best not being taken personally. To laugh, become embarrassed, or become angry may only prove to encourage the poor behavior.

Egocentricity

Many people who experience a brain injury display a childlike egocentricity. This is the result of frontal lobe damage. They do not consider the feelings of others around them and often are incapable of appreciating the needs of their family and friends. This is exhibited through demanding and unreasonable behavior, wanting every moment of their caregiver's time and attention, and a complete lack of gratitude for the enormous efforts and sacrifices made by their family on their behalf (Winslade, 1998). Self-centeredness is the source of many relationship difficulties following a brain injury. Ponsford (2013) describes the tendency to develop ways of attracting attention such as joking, clowning around, constant demands for forms of assistance, swearing, becoming physically aggressive, or engaging in self-abusive behaviors. The other aspect of egocentricity is the proclivity toward dependence. The survivor of a brain injury can become very dependent on those who are caring for him/her. Total dependency is difficult to sustain and not encouraged. Some caregivers believe that the process of recovery further exacerbates the egocentricity because all efforts are aimed at the survivor. The survivor becoming aware of others in the family is a process that accompanies longer term recovery.

Managing Egocentricity

One of the strongest deterrents to manage self-centeredness is to withdraw attention. Inappropriate behavior is meant to attract the attention of their caregiver. However, it is unhealthy and often dangerous. It is recommended that the family member or caregiver, after surveying the situation to ensure the survivor of brain injury is safe and is not in genuine need of help, ignore the behavior. By reacting, either positively or negatively, "one is reinforcing the behaviour by giving the TBI person what they want most, namely attention" (Ponsford, 2013). Of course, reinforcing appropriate behavior with a reward or attention will help shape the survivor to act appropriately.

Not allowing the survivor to be manipulative requires a set of consistent rules. Bargaining or threatening is discouraged. Joel suffered a severe TBI at the age of 17 in a car accident. His mom, Claire, was a neuropsychologist with a local private university. Joel became demanding and threatened to bang his head into a wall if his mom did not discharge him from rehabilitation. Her response? "Joel, I don't negotiate with terrorists." She turned around and left. He got the message. She would not allow herself to be manipulated with his threat of self-harm, and he finished his rehabilitation. He and his mom are doing well as of this writing. After treatment, he was accepted to a university and is active in a social service fraternity, while working on an accounting degree.

Conclusion

The cognitive deficits of brain injury are one of the invisible aspects of the disability. This chapter described the attention, concentration, awareness, memory, disinhibition, egocentrism, and processing and understanding deficits, along with the various ways to manage these issues in the recovery process. Hopefully, understanding the origin and the progression of cognitive deficits will shed light on the difficulty families have in navigating such behaviors. Implementation of some of the compensatory strategies will help the survivor to create management skills toward cognitive and behavioral improvements. Cognitive rehabilitation therapy and metacognition strategy instruction were highlighted as effective techniques to improve cognitive function after a brain injury. The next chapter addresses the prevalence and treatment of depression and anxiety.

References

Allen, C., & Ruff, R. (1990). Self-ratings versus neuropsychological performance of moderate versus severe head-injured patients. *Brain Injury*, *4*, 7–17.

Bandura, A. (1989). Regulation of cognitive processes through perceived self-efficacy. *Developmental Psychology*, *25*, 729–735.

Barman, A., Chatterjee, A., & Bhide, R. (2016). Cognitive impairment and rehabilitation strategies after traumatic brain injury. *Indian Journal of Psychological Medicine*, *38*(3), 172–181. https://doi.org/10.4103/0253-7176.183086

Chiaravalloti, N., Dobryakova, E., Wylie, G., & DeLuca, J. (2015). Examining the efficacy of the modified story memory technique (mSMT) in persons with TBI using functional magnetic resonance imaging (fMRI): The TBI-MEM trial. *Journal of Head Trauma Rehabilitation*, *30*(4), 261–269.

Cicerone, K. (1996). Attention deficits and dual task demands after mild traumatic brain injury. *Brain Injury*, *10*(2), 79–89.

Copley, A., Smith, K., Savill, K., & Finch, E. (2015). Does metacognition strategy instruction improve impaired receptive cognitive-communication skills following acquired brain injury? *Brain Injury, 29*(11), 1309–1316. https://doi.org/10.3109/02699052.2015.1043343

Crosson, B., Barco, P., Velozo, C., Bolesta, M., Cooper, P., Werts, D., & Brobeck, T. (1989). Awareness and compensation in postacute head injury rehabilitation. *Journal of Head Trauma Rehabilitation, 4*(3), 46–54. https://doi.org/10.1097/00001199-198909000-00008

Dirette, D. (2002). The development of awareness and the use of compensatory strategies for cognitive deficits. *Brain Injury, 16*(10), 861–871. https://doi.org/10.1080/02699050210131902

Eckert, M., Menon, V., Walczak, A., Ahlstrom, J., Denslow, S., Horwitz, A., & Dubno, J. (2009). At the heart of the ventral attention system: The right anterior insula. *Human Brain Mapping, 30*(8), 2530–2541. https://doi.org/10.1002/hbm.20688

Fleming, J., & Strong, J. (1995). Self-awareness of deficits following acquired brain injury: Considerations for rehabilitation. *British Journal of Occupational Therapy, 58*, 55–60.

Gasquoine, P. (1992). Affective state and awareness of sensory and cognitive effects after closed head injury. *Neuropsychology, 6*, 187–196.

Gronwall, D., Wrightson, P., & Waddell, P. (1998). *Head injury: The facts* (2nd ed.). Oxford University Press.

Himanen, L., Portin, R., Tenovuo, O., Taiminen, T., Koponen, S., Hiekkanen, H., & Helenius, H. (2009). Attention and depressive symptoms in chronic phase after traumatic brain injury. *Brain Injury, 23*(3), 220–227. https://doi.org/10.1080/02699050902748323

Kennedy, M., Coelho, C., Turkstra, L., Ylvisaker, M., Sohlberg, M., Yorkston, K., Chiou, H., & Kan, P. (2008). Intervention for executive functions after traumatic brain injury: A systematic review, meta-analysis and clinical recommendations. *Neuropsychological Rehabilitation, 18*(3), 257–299. https://doi.org/10.1080/09602010701748644

Kit, K., Mateer, C., & Graves, R. (2007). The influence of memory beliefs in individuals with traumatic brain injury. *Rehabilitation Psychology, 52*(1), 25–32. https://doi.org/10.1037/0090-5550.52.1.25

Knutson, K., Dal Monte, O., Schintu, S., Wassermann, E., Raymont, V., Grafman, J., & Krueger, F. (2015). Areas of brain damage underlying increased reports of behavioral disinhibition. *Journal of Neuropsychiatry and Clinical Neurosciences, 27*(3), 193–198. https://doi.org/10.1176/appi.neuropsych.14060126

Lezak, M. (1982). The problem of assessing executive functions. *International Journal of Psychology, 17*(1–4), 281–297.

Lezak, M. (1988). Brain damage is a family affair. *Journal of Clinical and Experimental Neuropsychology, 10*, 111–123.

Malouf, T., Langdon, R., & Taylor, A. (2014). The insight interview: A new tool for measuring deficits in awareness after traumatic brain injury. *Brain Injury, 28*(12), 1523–1541. https://doi.org/10.3109/02699052.2014.922700

Niemann, H., Ruff, R., & Kramer, J. (1996). An attempt towards differentiating attentional deficits in traumatic brain injury. *Neuropsychology Review, 6*, 11–46. https://link.springer.com/article/10.1007/BF01875418

Ponsford, J. (2013). Assessment and management of behaviour problems. In J. Ponsford, S. Sloan, & P. Snow (Eds.), *Traumatic brain injury: Rehabilitation for everyday adaptive living* (2nd ed., pp. 164–191). Psychology Press.

Rath, J., Hennessy, J., & Diller, L. (2003). Social problem solving and community integration in postacute rehabilitation outpatients with traumatic brain injury. *Rehabilitation Psychology, 48*(3), 137–144. https://doi.org/10.1037/0090-5550.48.3.137

Rees, L., Marshall, S., Hartridge, C., Mackie, D., & Weiser, M. for the Erabi Group (2007). Cognitive interventions post acquired brain injury. *Brain Injury, 21*(2), 161–200. https://doi.org/10.1080/02699050701201813

Richardson, C., McKay, A., & Ponsford, J. (2014). The trajectory of awareness across the first year after traumatic brain injury: The role of biopsychosocial factors. *Brain Injury, 28*(13–14), 1711–1720. https://doi.org/10.3109/02699052.2014.954270

Saux, G., Demey, I., Rojas, G., & Feldberg, C. (2014). Cognitive rehabilitation therapy after acquired brain injury in Argentina: Psychosocial outcomes in connection with the time elapsed before treatment initiation. *Brain Injury, 28*(11), 1447–1454. https://doi.org/10.3109/02699052.2014.919528

Sohlberg, M., & Mateer, C. (1987). Effectiveness of an attention-training program. *Journal of Clinical and Experimental Neuropsychology, 9*(2), 117–130. https://doi.org/10.1080/01688638708405352

Stratton, M., & Gregory, R. (1994). After traumatic brain injury: A discussion of consequences. *Brain Injury, 8*(7), 631–645.

Tsaousides, T., & Gordon, W. (2009). Cognitive rehabilitation following traumatic brain injury: Assessment to treatment. *Mount Sinai Journal of Medicine: A Journal of Transitional and Personalized Medicine, 76*(2), 173–181.

Verfaellie, M., Amick, M., & Vasterling, J. (2012). Effects of traumatic brain injury – Associated neurocognitive alterations on posttraumatic stress disorder. In J. Vasterling, R. Bryant, & T. Keane (Eds.), *PTSD and mild traumatic brain injury* (pp. 82–102). The Guilford Press.

von Cramon, D., & Matthes-von Cramon, G. (1992). Reflections on the treatment of brain-injured patients suffering from problem solving disorders. *Neuropsychological Rehabilitation, 2*, 207–229.

Wallace, C., & Bogner, J. (2000). Awareness of deficits: Emotional implications for persons with brain injury and their significant others. *Brain Injury, 14*(6), 549–562. https://doi.org/10.1080/026990500120457

Winslade, W. (1998). *Confronting traumatic brain injury: Devastation, hope, and healing*. Yale University Press.

8 Counseling Depression and Anxiety

Case Study

A Massachusetts Institute of Technology (MIT) graduate with two master's degrees, John was referred to counseling by his neuropsychologist due to ongoing anxiety and chronic depression. At age 48, John was at the top of his game as an executive with an international banking company. Numbers were his passion, yet after suffering a mild traumatic brain injury (mTBI) from a car accident two years prior, he could no longer solve mathematical problems or balance a checkbook. He did not recognize himself and was concerned that he would be unable to return to a vocation he very much enjoyed. No longer able to read a spreadsheet or process the complex issues that stem from multilevel calculations, John took a leave of absence from his work. Adding to his depression and anxiety was the knowledge that he was the major financial contributor to both his household and that of his parents. He also supported his daughter at university.

During the initial evaluation with his therapist, John shared the neuropsychological determination of post-concussive syndrome, major depressive disorder, and general anxiety disorder. John reported light and sound sensitivity, extreme fatigue, frequent headaches, slowed processing, low-grade depression, and anxiety, which was especially pronounced at work. John was worried about his future ability to support not only his family but also his aging parents, who lived next door to him and his wife, Louise. John's daughter was away at college when the injury occurred. Prior to the wreck, John was active in his church and participated in weekly game nights with his neighborhood friends.

During a couples session, John shared that he was currently experiencing multiple physical and cognitive problems from the collision. He stated that he was working with a physiatrist, a physical therapist, a speech therapist, and now a psychotherapist. The emotional symptoms appeared to stem from the mTBI because he did not exhibit such symptoms before the accident. The therapist requested testing records from the neuropsychologist. She also discussed the process of psychotherapy and what to expect. Therapeutic goals were established: (1) brain injury education, (2) development of compensatory strategies for the deficits from the mTBI, (3) anxiety management, (4) reduction of depressive symptoms, (5) refer to psychiatrist for medication consultation, and (6) development of return-to-work criteria.

DOI: 10.4324/9781003301912-8

John participated actively in treatment and was able to acknowledge that the deficits from the mTBI contributed to his depression and anxiety. The frequency of sessions initially was weekly, and as he progressed, the sessions decreased to two times per month, then stretched to monthly. Occasionally his wife would join in the sessions to offer observations that she had made at home. Interestingly, Louise was a mental health counselor and was able to recognize the depressive and anxious symptoms. She readily learned about mTBI and the cognitive and emotional deficits that accompany the diagnosis. Her accommodation was invaluable for John and his recovery.

A strength of the counseling process for John was to identify that his symptoms could be managed through various coping strategies. Additionally, he appreciated the biblical influence of how to manage depression and anxiety with specific truths from the scripture. The counselor was able to help him recognize what symptom originated from what disorder or deficit. For example, his anxiety stemmed from the fear of not being able to provide for his family or return to work. Depression came from his feeling of not being in control and not knowing what his future capabilities would encompass. John found comfort in the passage from Matthew 11:28 (NIV): "Come to me, all you who are weary and burdened, and I will give you rest." Managing his fatigue reduced his other physical symptoms and decreased his anxiety and depression. Another comforting passage was Romans 11:29 (NIV): "For God's gifts and his call are irrevocable." This promise helped John to recognize that he would be able to return to finance in some form.

During the 18 months of counseling, John was able to practice compensatory strategies to manage his deficits from the brain injury and his emotional challenges. The counselor composed a letter to his employer identifying accommodations needed for John to make a successful return to work. These considerations included the following: (1) allow for frequent and extended breaks, (2) provide a private or separate office away from foot traffic, (3) give instruction in verbal and written format, (4) provide the ability to reduce lighting in his office, (5) provide an augmented computer screen to manage brightness, and (6) provide the ability to work from home part of the week. John's company employed these accommodations, and eventually he was able to return to full-time work. Although John continued to struggle with headaches and sensory issues, he was able to employ his strategies as needed. He reported residual anxiety that came from adjusting to a new normal. John stated that he did not feel depressed. His treatment team and family all worked together to ensure a successful recovery and return to work. Although John does not work at the same pace that he did prior to the car wreck, he reports feeling happier and likes who he has become.

After returning to work full time, John was given the opportunity to work with a nutritionist. He believed that losing weight would give him more energy and flexibility and improve his conditioning. John committed to the program, which included "clean eating," weighing his food, and measuring his intake. He began walking daily with his wife. After one year of the new eating routine and exercise, John had lost over 50 pounds. He stated that he feels better than he ever has in his life. John believes that the nutrition changes contributed to a better quality of life. He states that he feels completely healed from his mTBI and is enjoying life and taking care of his parents and his family. John was promoted back to the same position he enjoyed before his injury.

Depression and Anxiety Overview

Psychological reactions to traumatic brain injury (TBI) are varied and complex. Of mood disorders, depression and anxiety are the most frequently reported. Jorge (2008) stated that mood disturbances affecting brain injury survivors and family members have a large impact on family relationships, social integration, and return to productive activity. Douglas and Spellacy (2000) reported that previous studies indicated that at least one-half of adults with severe TBI as well as their primary caregivers experienced depression and anxiety. Unfortunately, one-half of the survivors studied reported that the significant levels of depression did not dissipate over time. However, they noted that social support in the form of community, social network, intimate, and confiding relationships met the long-term needs of survivors and caregivers. Awareness of the impact of the brain injury often creates feelings of despondency and anxiety. Recognition of these mood disturbances as a normal response to recovery allows the rehabilitation to proceed in a positive manner (Gronwall et al., 1998). Treatment of these mood disorders is vitally important as they can have long-lasting effects on both quality of life and subjective cognitive status up to ten years post-injury (McIntyre et al., 2020).

Major Depressive Disorder

Although there are a wide range of reports of depression after brain injury, Ashman and colleagues estimate that 42–53% of individuals experience a depressive disorder episode in the first year post-injury (Ashman et. al., 2014). They reported that even the most conservative estimates of depression place survivors of brain injury at higher risk for developing the mood disorder than the general population. Stress and allostatic load, a concept referring to the long-lasting effects of persistently activated stress reactions, have been linked to the development of depression post-TBI (McIntyre et al., 2020). Hawthorne et al. (2009) concluded that survivors of TBI

> experienced worse general health, elevated probabilities of depression, social isolation and worse labor force participation rate . . . and unless treatment includes targeting services at those areas of life identified in this and other studies, limited outcomes can be expected.

Therefore, early identification of those at risk for posttraumatic depression and the development of effective prevention and treatment could improve the long-term outcomes for survivors of TBI (Juengst et al., 2015).

There are, however, challenges in the diagnosis of depression with brain injury. Some symptoms mimic the sequelae of TBI, such as fatigue, cognitive deficits, and sleep impairment (Dyer et al., 2016). Depressive disorders manifest as changes in mood, behavior, and thinking. Some of the mood changes are sadness, tearfulness, agitation, and irritability. Examples of behavior alterations are psychomotor retardation, social withdrawal, poor hygiene, and lack of motivation. Common cognitive changes are helplessness, hopelessness, self-criticism, indecisiveness, and loss of interest. Depressive symptoms specific to brain injury are sleep difficulties, impaired judgment, loss of purpose, poor concentration, and poor emotional control.

Another challenge for diagnosis is the variance in reports between the survivor of TBI and his/her family members. The parent or caregiver may report that his/her loved one cries daily, but the survivor may report feeling "a little sad." Other clients may present incongruently, saying they are depressed while bearing a smile. Awareness or lack of awareness complicates the issue as well. In those cases, observation and family member reports provide a more definitive diagnosis.

An important distinction to consider is that depression can be a natural occurrence as the survivor of brain injury recovers and becomes more aware of his/her losses and deficits from the injury. For example, a newly diagnosed survivor may not have awareness of the injury or of its effects. However, as recovery continues, the survivor will recognize that there are limitations to his/her activities, loss of independence, loss of his/her former self, impaired ability to think or function, and changes in his/her social and family relationships. Once the survivor becomes aware of the deficits from the injury, depressive symptoms often emerge. The mood of despondency may come and go over days, weeks, or months. In this case, depression is associated with ambiguous grief and, therefore, could be considered reactive depression. Although the depression from the increased awareness is concerning, it is also important to acknowledge it as a stage of recovery and not necessarily a permanent mental health diagnosis.

The *Diagnostic and Statistical Manual of Mental Disorders, Fifth Edition* (DSM-V; American Psychiatric Association (APA), 2013) states that the presence of a depressed mood or loss of interest for at least two weeks with the addition of at least five of the following symptoms meets the criteria for Major Depressive Disorder. The symptoms include the following: (1) depressed mood most of the day, nearly every day, (2) diminished interest or pleasure in all, or almost all, activities, (3) significant weight loss or weight gain, (4) insomnia or hypersomnia, (5) psychomotor retardation or agitation, (6) fatigue or loss of energy, (7) feelings of worthlessness or inappropriate guilt, (8) reduced ability to think or concentrate or indecisiveness, and (9) recurrent thoughts of death or suicidal ideation, with or without a plan.

Social support made a significant impact on lowering depression in survivors of TBI. Previous research demonstrated that the lack of social contact remained a permanent, long-term outcome for this population. Tomberg et al. (2005)

studied a group of survivors of TBI from Estonia, a post-Socialist country. The study demonstrated that the presence of individuals who were able to consistently provide care, help, trust, and emotional support remained essential for long-term rehabilitation. In their study, the support mainly came from family members, while the number of nonrelatives among the supporters was significantly lower. A poorer support system, indicative of an inadequate or malfunctioning supporters' network, made more difference than the number of supporters. Hoofien et al. (2001) reported that 31% of survivors of TBI had no friends outside their family. Loss of social contact, difficulty making new friends, and misinterpretation of social cues characterized poor social functioning.

Counseling Considerations

Risk assessment and risk management are the first line of defense when working with clients who experience depression. Unfortunately, suicidal ideations and suicide attempts are three to four times higher in the TBI population than in the general population (Ponsford et al., 2013). Risk assessment includes asking the client the following questions: does s/he have thoughts of hurting him/herself; does s/he have a history of self-harm; does s/he have a plan to hurt him/herself; and, if so, does s/he have the means to execute the plan. Affirmative responses require referral to an inpatient psychiatric facility or emergency department for emergent care or to a psychiatrist who can provide a medication consultation. It is preferred that a trusted family member accompany his/her loved one to an emergent appointment.

To date, there have been limited psychotherapeutic trials targeting depression with the TBI population. However, there are trends reporting therapy modalities such as cognitive-behavioral therapy, education, family education, and support groups as being effective in successfully treating depression (Marsh et al., 2002). In 2004, the World Health Organization and US Department of Defense published a manual titled *Rehabilitation for Persons with Traumatic Brain Injury* (World Health Organization, Disability and Rehabilitation Team, United States, Department of Defense & Drucker Brain Injury Center, 2004). The manual states that an important role of a healthcare professional is to "help the person, family and community to understand all disabilities from brain injury, and to learn how to assist an injured person to recover as many abilities as possible." Because each survivor presents a wide range of depressive triggers, Ruff and Chester (2014) recommend that the clinician should delineate the biopsychosocial stressors and specifically examine the extent to which each contributes to the overall depression of the client. Ashley and Connors (2010) have said that professionals working with TBI need to keep abreast of current research findings. They stressed the importance of having a broad knowledge of TBI and the ability to access a cadre of specialists associated with TBI recovery, because "knowledge is not widely distributed around the general medical community, and most practitioners have very little experience with this unique population" (Ashley & Connors, 2010).

Cognitive-Behavioral Therapy

One of the most prevalent and well-researched therapies for depression in the general population is cognitive-behavioral therapy (CBT). This approach is also well suited for survivors of TBI because it provides structure that reduces organizational demands and it provides learning and memory strategies, such as handouts, repetition, checklists, and thought logs (Ashman et al., 2014). Generally, CBT addresses issues associated with TBI such as depression, anger management, suicide prevention, low self-esteem, and anxiety management. Ponsford (2013) stated that CBT for depressed individuals post-TBI helps them to "understand the link between thoughts and their emotions." Ponsford recommended adaptations to CBT for the brain-injured population due to their cognitive impairments in the "domains of attention, memory, and executive function, which may limit their capacity to understand CBT concepts and absorb, retain, and carry over the ideas and strategies for addressing their psychological problems." These adaptions include "incorporating simplified concepts, concrete behavioral examples, pictorial handouts and cues, and considerable repetition, as well as booster sessions" (Ponsford, 2013). Therapeutic assistance may also be given to help the survivor of TBI to see the differences between their post-injury self and their pre-injury self in a more positive light and to begin to measure him/herself by what s/he has achieved post-injury (Ponsford, 2013). Further recommendations were the development of coping strategies such as "solving problems, working hard, using humour [and] physical recreation and seeking relaxing diversions" (Ponsford, 2013). An interesting outcome of the study was the finding that cognitive impairment was "not a barrier to achieving symptom reduction using [a] CBT protocol modified for this population" (Ponsford, 2013). Ashman and colleagues (2014) incorporated CBT in their study of 77 survivors of TBI with a diagnosis of depression. The techniques used included cognitive restructuring, which challenges and reshapes automatic thoughts into more rational self-statements; guided self-dialogue, which assists in generating more positive self-statements; mastery and planning to improve social outreach; and relaxation techniques to manage overwhelming emotions. At the end of their treatment, 35% of the participants reported that they were no longer depressed. Individual CBT counseling is recommended over group interventions because it can be tailored to meet the needs and issues of clients with TBI (Ponsford, 2013).

Psychotherapy

Despite the range of clinical evidence demonstrating the efficacy of psychotherapy with survivors of brain injury, the provision of these services remains scarce (Judd & Wilson, 2005). Neurologically oriented clinicians may have "over-estimated the differences between brain injured and non-brain injured individuals whilst under-estimating the extent to which the brain injury survivor has to cope with the same psychological issues as everyone else" (Judd &

Wilson, 2005). The balance between understanding brain injury and depression in light of one another is paramount to being effective as a counselor.

Broadly speaking, psychotherapy is a joint enterprise between a therapist and an individual to help him/her reduce distress and improve life satisfaction through changing thoughts, feelings, and behaviors. It is a collaborative effort, a working alliance toward agreed-upon goals based on trust, respect, understanding, and theoretical orientation. Fundamental aspects of psychotherapy represent several variables that operate at the same time. Six facets of psychotherapy include "therapeutic contract, therapeutic operations, the therapeutic bond, self-relatedness, in-session impacts, and the phases of treatment made up of sequential events within and also between psychotherapy consultations" (Coetzer, 2010). Different reports have commented that the psychotherapeutic approach is limited in scope with the brain injury population due to "reduced self-awareness (or insight), memory impairment, and executive control impairment" (Coetzer, 2010). However, Coetzer recognized Prigitano's work, which stated that there are four components to the psychological management of individuals with TBI. These components are "reinforcement of desirable behaviours, ensuring that the patient is provided with adequate information, helping the person develop self-awareness, and, finally, nurturing and using the therapeutic relationship to help the patient make more effective or functional choices" (Coetzer, 2010). The counseling process can come with great strains "due to the complex inter-play between organic and psychological damage and the resulting range of sequelae which the survivor and the therapist will have to engage with" (Judd & Wilson, 2005). It is helpful to acknowledge which symptoms are due to brain injury versus those due to depression. In the counseling process, clients become better able to manage the symptoms with more efficiency if they are aware of the origin of that symptom.

Understanding the organicity of brain damage is crucial in assisting the survivor of brain injury and his/her family. The second most important aspect of counseling is learning how the brain injury has affected the specific client. It is commonly said in the brain injury community, "if you've seen one brain injury; you've seen one brain injury." It is also essential to understand the meaning the client gives to his/her injury, who his/her post-injury self is, and the psychosocial consequences of his/her brain injury deficits (Judd & Wilson, 2005).

Considerations for the brain-injured population include adjusting the length of sessions to accommodate attention challenges and fatigue; offering written handouts of strategies discussed; summarizing the session in written format to give to the client during the session or to send through email; reducing sensory input in the counseling office, such as use of dimmed lighting and noise-cancelling machines; and using repetition as needed. Ronald Ruff and his colleagues (2016) offer a four-step treatment process for psychotherapy with survivors of brain injury:

- Assess the client's overall energy level.
- Address issues of anger, depression, and anxiety.

- Encourage the client to accept his/her new status as it relates to future gains and that return to a pre-morbid state is not reasonable
- Assist the client to find purpose.

Finding purpose includes the client grieving the loss of his/her former self and creating future goals that are meaningful (Ruff et al., 2016). Krych and Schmidt (2015) believe that "it is absolutely critical that [clinicians] properly prepare those we work with for a lifelong process of re-creating their lives, finding joy and meaningfulness, and seeking what they need." Additionally, they believe that part of the role of the therapist working with a survivor of TBI is "to develop an outlook and behavior that reflects the possibilities for life after brain injury" (Krych & Schmidt, 2015). Coetzer (2010) reported that clients identified that the "clinician's listening skills can play an important role in helping with exploring, expressing, and understanding the losses and grief that can accompany brain injury." He also supports the "development of a robust therapeutic relationship, providing longer-term follow-up and easy access to the therapist during crises and relapses." Overall, the psychotherapeutic therapy model incorporates a healthy therapeutic relationship, and from that place, insight and awareness along with coping strategies can be developed and implemented.

Christian Counseling

The role of a Christian counselor is to comfort, educate, equip, and encourage each survivor of TBI utilizing the tenets of the Christian faith. To create coping strategies, instill hope for healing and recovery, and journey with survivors through the grieving of their pre-injury functioning and encouraging them toward post-injury quality of life are the overall goals. Innate in this approach is the belief that God is intricately involved in the recovery process. Because people are made in the image of God, the *imago Dei*, He is inherently invested in their becoming the best they can be, despite and during affliction.

The term "depression" is not found in the original scripture. However, it is described throughout the scripture with words or phrases such as downcast, discouraged, downhearted, troubled, despairing, brokenhearted, miserable, or weakened spirit. King David cried in Psalm 42:3 (NIV), "My tears are my food both day and night." He says in Psalm 6:6 (NIV), "I am worn out from my groaning. All night long I flood my bed with weeping and drench my couch with tears." Despondent, Elijah told God, "I have had enough, Lord . . . Take my life; I am no better than my ancestors." after being threatened by Queen Jezebel (1 Kings 19:4, NIV). Depression can be a normal human experience in the face of adversity. For survivors of brain injury and their family members, it is a common experience as they come to understand the deficits resulting from the injury and attempt to move toward acceptance and the creation of coping strategies. During times of depression, it is not uncommon for a survivor to say s/he cannot pray or feel a connection to God. It is in these times that it is helpful to remember Luke 5:20 (NIV), which says that "when Jesus saw their faith, he said 'Friend, your sins are forgiven.'" Jesus healed a man, not because of his own faith but because of the faith of his friends. There are times that, as individuals, it is difficult to drum up enough faith to go the Savior. Christian counselors have the holy opportunity to pray for their clients. Diane Landberg, PhD (2014), stated that it is possible that God allows counselors to see and hear things to pray for their clients and that the process of interceding brings God's purpose and order into their world. Similarly, when depression hits and depletes one's hope, it is important for the Christian counselor to express his/her hope for the client. "If you have run out of hope, please borrow some of mine." This is a statement that enlightens and encourages the client. One of the characteristics of the depression of survivors of TBI is fatigue. Jesus offers help with this issue in Matthew 11:28–30 (NIV):

> Come to me, all you who are weary and burdened, and I will give you rest. Take my yoke upon you and learn from me, for I am gentle and humble in heart, and you will find rest for your souls. For my yoke is easy and my burden is light.

Utilization of scriptural references to specific deficits from brain injury, including depression, is a well-placed help in the counseling process.

Faith Alternatives

Counselors who understand their client's worldview, which includes the person's religious belief systems or non-faith belief systems, will work most effectively with him/her. Belief systems outside of the Christian purview access faith and hope. Meaning and purpose are also sources of spirituality (Jones et al., 2018). The role of hope is important in successful therapeutic alliances. The survivors of brain injury need the sense of hope in themselves and in their therapist. Klonoff (1997) stated that clients are "perceptive; they sense if the therapist feels discouraged or disenchanted with the patient and his or her prognosis." By the nature of brain injury, many survivors of severe TBI have had near-death experiences. Those affected "may draw upon spiritual sources of meaning, comfort and strength as they adjust to their new circumstances and live with the long-term consequences of their illness or injury" (Jones et al., 2018). Koenig (2012) found that, in most studies, spirituality and religion were significantly associated with positive emotions, greater social support, and lower levels of depression, suicide, and anxiety. Jones et al. (2018) found that a connection to a higher power was a significant predictor of life satisfaction, reduced global stress, improved health perception, and patient competency. Johnstone et al. (2009) stated that survivors of TBI may expect to live decades post-injury and "may use religious and spiritual resources to help them cope with their disability, give new meaning to their lives based on their newly acquired disabilities and help them establish new life goals."

There is a distinction between religious well-being and existential well-being. Waldron-Perrine et al. (2011) explained that, "religious well-being refers specifically to a meaningful relationship with God, whereas existential well-being refers to the general belief that one's life is meaningful or has purpose." Spirituality can be separate from religious beliefs. Counselors should encourage clients to practice their spirituality or beliefs consistent with their moral standards as a means of mitigating depression, as this can be very helpful. Prayer, community contact in a synagogue or other place of worship, nature walks, and the search for one's sense of self and purpose are all activities that lend themselves to improved mood. A feeling of being connected and close to people one loves is predictive of improved health outcomes of depression. The perception of being cared for can also extend to the relationship with God or another higher power (Waldron-Perrine et al., 2011).

NON-FAITH ALTERNATIVES

General recommendations for clients with brain injury include physical accommodations and emotional and cognitive adjustments. While counseling a survivor of TBI, it may be helpful to refer the client to his/her primary physician to address any health concerns that proper nutrition and supplements may improve. Sitting outside in the sun or exposure to sunlight for at least 10–15 minutes per day helps to heal the body and brain. So that the client receives the full benefit, discourage the use of sunglasses. The healing blue and red rays of the sun need to travel through the retina to get to the brain. Another recommendation is for the client to walk for five to ten minutes each day. Physical movement helps improve balance and perspective. The creation of a safe space to journal or practice art or listen to music can also be helpful. The goal is to engage in self-nurturing behaviors. Normally, depression makes one focus on the negative and hopelessness or helplessness. Art is about creating, which fights the negative focus. It is important to adjust one's expectations to fit within the emotional energy of each given moment. Often, survivors of TBI tend to be self-critical, which creates more negativity. If s/he is able to adjusting his/her expectations from what s/he should be able to do to what s/he can do with the resources available, it will help him/her to create and sustain progress. The intentional reframing of disability to ability, what one can do, can be a helpful paradigm shift as well.

Generalized Anxiety Disorder

Generalized Anxiety Disorder (GAD) is part of the Anxiety Disorders spectrum according to the *Diagnostic and Statistical Manual of Mental Disorders, Fifth Edition* (DSM-V; APA, 2013). Anxiety is the most commonly occurring co-morbidity with depression. GAD is characterized by at least six months of excessive worry and anxiety. Albrecht et al. (2017) found that the prevalence of anxiety in survivors of TBI ranged between 10% and 33%. Someone diagnosed with GAD finds it difficult to control his/her worry and experiences significant distress in social, occupational, and family functioning. Additional symptoms include (1) restlessness or feeling on edge, (2) being easily fatigued, (3) difficulty concentrating or experiencing one's mind going blank, (4) irritability, and (5) sleep disturbance (APA, 2013). For an accurate diagnosis, it is necessary for the clinician to assess the presence of a relationship between the onset, exacerbation, or remission of the general medical condition and the anxiety symptoms. As noted earlier, depression and anxiety are associated with the brain injury survivor's loss of independence, loss of self, and loss of prior level of functioning. Coetzer (2010) stated that one of the psychological concepts of GAD relevant to survivors of TBI is the issue of control. The cognitive impairments contribute to a "reduced ability to control the environments or to solve problems that may have appeared straightforward or even trivial to deal with in the past" (Coetzer, 2010). Additionally, some of the physical symptoms of brain injury, such as dizziness, tremors, or sleep disturbance, may contribute to anxiety for the survivor. Coetzer (2010) differentiates the symptoms that are specific to TBI but not necessarily to GAD. These include (1) realistic worries about the future in response to the TBI, (2) fatigue and poor concentration, and (3) irritability. Interestingly, Ponsford et al. (2020) found that older age was associated with a reduction in anxiety symptomology.

Counseling Considerations

There are several approaches to managing the symptoms of GAD for survivors of brain injury. Muscle relaxation, biofeedback, visual imagery, and cognitive restructuring may be used to decrease the symptoms. Ponsford (2013) emphasizes coping strategies such as problem-solving, developing a positive outlook, and utilizing humor as helpful for reducing anxiety. She also believes that reassuring the client that s/he is not going mad or losing his/her mind is an important strategy for dealing with chronic anxiety. Coetzer (2010) identifies the following psychological interventions to effectively treat GAD: (1) reassurance and information, (2) supportive psychotherapy, (3) cognitive-behavioral therapy, and (4) mindfulness. Recognizing the client's worries and allowing him/her to voice those worries are considered the first step toward understanding the underlying issues fueling his/her anxieties. If low self-confidence is a factor in anxiety, cognitive-behavioral methods are particularly useful (Coetzer, 2010). Assisting the client to identify possible cognitive distortions coupled with assigning a behavioral task that can be successfully implemented provides a positive experience. Additionally, it is imperative to assist the client toward hopeful outcomes. When working with survivors of brain injury who struggle with anxiety, it is important to assist them to pursue their personal goals.

Christian Counseling

With brain injury, anxiety comes in the form of free-floating worries about the individual's current level of functioning and the fear that s/he may not be able to return to his/her pre-injury level of functioning. A key to helping these individuals lies in identifying the truth in their recovery process. The scripture says that Jesus is "the way, the truth, and the life" (John 14:6, NIV). Because the nature of anxiety is fear, it is important to help the client recognize what is true. This is a means of reducing the fear, the "what-if" kind of thinking that exacerbates anxiety. Replacement of "what if" with "what is true" is key to the client grounding him/herself. This technique helps the client to concentrate on what is true in the moment, with statements such as "I am safe. I am loved." An additional grounding technique is to tune into one's surroundings. Ask the client to share what s/he is seeing, hearing, and feeling. These questions help the client to recognize what is true now.

There are several biblical references that address the role of anxiety in one's life and how to manage it successfully. Philippians 4:6–7 is one of the most recited scriptures about anxiety. The Message version says,

> [D]on't fret or worry. Instead of worrying, pray. Let the petitions and praises shape your worries into prayers, letting God know your concerns. Before you know it, a sense of God's wholeness, everything coming together for good, will come and settle you down. It's wonderful what happens when Christ displaces worry at the center of your life.

1 Peter 5:7 (New American Standard Bible, NASB) advises: "[C]ast all your anxiety on Him, because He cares about you." Proverbs 12:25 (NASB) says that, "[A]nxiety in a person's heart weighs it down. But a good word makes it glad." Finally, Matthew 6:25 (NASB) offers this as a means of managing anxiety:

> For this reason I say to you, do not be worried about your life, as to what you will eat or what you will drink; nor for your body, as what you will put on. Is life not more than food, and the body more than clothing?

Another key to managing anxiety is to concentrate on peace and safety. Psalm 91:1,2 (NIV) reminds the reader that, "[W]hoever dwells in the shelter of the Most High will rest in the shadow of the Almighty. I will say of the Lord, 'He is my refuge and my fortress, my God, in whom I trust.'" Faith in God's providence creates a sense of safety and peace for survivors of TBI and their family members. Isaiah 26:3 (New King James Version, NKJV) further underlines this belief with the following truth: "You will keep him in perfect peace, whose mind is stayed on You, because he trusts You." And in Romans 8:28 (NKJV), the Apostle Paul says, "And we know that all things work together for good to those who love God, to those who are the called according to His purpose." One survivor of TBI often says, "God's got this." This is her way of staying mindful that God has her best interest at heart and that He will see her through whatever difficulty. Last, 1 John 4:18 (NIV) says that "perfect love drives out all fear." In the Bible, God is perfect love. So, to help the client to focus on God and His character will eliminate his/her anxiety about the unknown.

Faith Alternatives

Imagery is an example of managing anxiety from a non-faith-based perspective. One client stated that he imagined his fear (anxiety/panic) as a monster at the end of a long hallway. He then imagined stairs to reduce the power of the monster. With every new way of managing the fear, he imagined a light switch that shed light on the menacing figure. Managing the fear was combating irrationality. Eventually, the client said that the monster reduced in size and his self-empowerment grew. He no longer believed the worst case but recognized the positive outcomes of a certain event.

To imagine anxiety as a signal or a spot on a map is another way of reframing the fear from oppressive to informative. For example, why is the anxiety happening now? What is the anxiety trying to say? What is the message? Often, fear needs an anchor to decrease. Free-floating anxiety is perpetuated by "why" questions. The anchor represents the truth in the present circumstance. Survivors of TBI question whether they will get better or whether the rest of their life will be like it is presently. It is helpful to remind them of the truth of science. Their progress is inevitable, barring another injury. Trust in the process requires patience and hope to thereby fight the fear and anxiety.

Square, or box, breathing has been suggested to help alleviate anxiety. Initially developed for first responders, this technique is meant to relieve stress in high-anxiety situations. There are four steps to the method: (1) inhale through the nose to the count of four, (2) hold the breath to the count of four, (3) exhale through the mouth to the count of four, and (4) hold the breath to the count of four. The person can repeat this four times. This technique is a model for practiced breathing that helps to relax the body and reduce the stress of the brain.

Conclusion

Mood disorders such as depression and anxiety are the most frequent psychiatric illnesses observed in survivors of TBI. Rush and her colleagues (2006) believe that these emotional disturbances may be due in part to "a disruption of affective brain systems and/or the stress of adjustment to post-injury environmental demands." Several therapy modalities have been employed to effectively treat depression and anxiety within the brain injury community. However, to date, none has been researched as the "gold standard" of treatment. Clinicians have utilized cognitive-behavioral therapy, psychotherapy, support groups, mindfulness, and family therapy with some degree of success. Faith-based counseling offers a unique approach that is well suited for survivors of TBI and their family members who verbalize a strong faith in God. In this chapter, specific methods and scriptures were given to address the depression and anxiety associated with brain injury. Encouragement was given for the clinician to incorporate these biblical truths into his/her therapy practice. Additionally, recognition of the role of spiritual health in the recovery process is thematic to the faith-based counseling perspective. Last, therapy techniques were presented for those who hold no faith belief or another faith-based belief system, such as imagery, nature walks, deep breathing, and journaling. The next chapter addresses the role of ambiguous grief in the recovery process.

References

Albrecht, J., Peters, M., Smith, G., & Rao, V. (2017). Anxiety and posttraumatic stress disorder among Medicare beneficiaries after traumatic brain injury. *Journal of Head Trauma Rehabilitation, 32*, 178–184.

American Psychiatric Association. (2013). *Diagnostic and statistical manual of mental disorders* (5th ed.).

Ashley, M., & Connors, S. (2010). Managing patients with traumatic brain injury: Across a long and often difficult continuum of care. *Care Management, 16*, 7–10.

Ashman, T., Cantor, J. B., Tsaousides, T., Spielman, L., & Gordon, W. (2014). Comparison of cognitive behavioral therapy and supportive psychotherapy for the treatment of depression following traumatic brain injury: A randomized controlled trial. *Journal of Head Trauma Rehabilitation, 29*(6), 467–478.

Coetzer, R. (2010). *Anxiety and mood disorders following traumatic brain injury: Clinical assessment and psychotherapy*. Routledge.

Douglas, J., & Spellacy, F. (2000). Correlates of depression in adults with severe traumatic brain injury and their carers. *Brain Injury, 14*, 71–88.

Dyer, J., Williams, R., Bombardier, C., Vannoy, S., & Fann, J. (2016). Evaluating the psychometric properties of 3 depression measures in a sample of persons with traumatic brain injury and major depressive disorder. *Journal of Head Trauma Rehabilitation, 31*(3), 225–232.

Gronwall, D., Wrightson, P., & Waddell, P. (1998). *Head injury: The facts* (2nd ed.). Oxford Press.

Hawthorne, G., Gruen, R., & Kaye, A. (2009). Traumatic brain injury and long-term quality of life: Findings from an Australian study. *Journal of Neurotrauma, 26*, 1623–1633.

Hoofien, D., Gilboa, A., Vakil, E., & Donovick, P. (2001). Traumatic brain injury (TBI) 10–20 years later: A comprehensive outcome study of psychiatric symptomology, cognitive abilities and psychosocial functioning. *Brain Injury, 15*, 189–209.

Johnstone, B., Yoon, D., Rupright, J., & Reid-Arndt, S. (2009). Relationships among spiritual beliefs, religious practices, congregational support and health for individuals with traumatic brain injury. *Brain Injury, 23*(5), 411–419. https://doi.org/10.1080/02699050902788501

Jones, K., Pryor, J., Care-Unger, C., & Simpson, G. (2018). Spirituality and its relationship with a positive adjustment following traumatic brain injury: A scoping review. *Brain Injury, 32*(13–14), 1612–1622. https://doi.org/10.1080/02699052.2018.1511066

Jorge, R.E. (2008). Mood and anxiety disorders following traumatic brain injury. *Psychiatric Times, 25*, 64–66.

Judd, D., & Wilson, S. (2005). Psychotherapy with brain injury survivors: An investigation of the challenges encountered by clinicians and their modifications to therapeutic practice. *Brain Injury 19*(6), 437–449. https://doi.org/10.1080/02699050400010994

Juengst, S., Kumar, R., Failla, M., Goyal A., & Wagner, A. K. (2015). Acute inflammatory biomarker profiles predict depression risk following moderate to severe traumatic brain injury. *Journal of Head Trauma Rehabilitation, 30*(3), 207–218.

Klonoff, P. (1997). Individual and group psychotherapy in milieu-oriented neurorehabilitation. *Applied Neuropsychology, 4*, 107–118.

Koenig, H. (2012). Religion, spirituality, and health: The research and clinical implications. *Psychiatry, 2012*, 1–33. https://doi.org/10.5402/2012/278730

Krych, D., & Schmidt, M.J. (2015). Beyond the evidence: What have we learned? Beyond the evidence: What do we believe? *Brain Injury Professional, 12*(1), 12–13.

Landberg, D. (2014). *In our lives first: Meditations for counselors*. Diane Langberg, PhD & Associates.

Marsh, N., Kersel, D., Havill, J., & Sleigh, J. (2002). Caregiver burden during the year following severe traumatic brain injury. *Journal of Clinical and Experimental Neuropsychology, 24*, 434–447.

McIntyre, A., Rice, D., Janzen, S., Mehta, S., Harnett, A., Caughlin, S., Sequeira, K., & Teasell, R. (2020). Anxiety, depression, and quality of life among subgroups of individuals with acquired brain injury: The role of anxiety sensitivity and experiential avoidance. *NeuroRehabilitation, 47*(1), 45–53.

Ponsford, J. (2013). Dealing with the impact of TBI on psychological adjustment and relationships. In J. Ponsford, S. Sloan, & P. Snow (Eds.), *Traumatic brain injury: Rehabilitation for everyday adaptive living* (2nd ed., pp. 226–262). Psychology Press.

Ponsford, J., Lee, N., Wong, D., McKay, A., Haines, K., Downing, M., Alway, Y., Furtado, C., & O'Donnell, M. (2020). Factors associated with response to adapted cognitive behavioral therapy for anxiety and depression following traumatic brain injury. *Journal of Head Trauma Rehabilitation, 35*(2), 117–126.

Ruff, R., & Chester, S. (2014). *Effective psychotherapy for individuals with brain injury*. Guilford Press.

Ruff, R., Blank, J., & Schraa, J. (2016). How can emotions be more effectively assessed in individuals with traumatic brain injury. *Brain Injury Professional, 13*(3), 18–21.

Rush, B., Malec, J., Brown, A., & Moessner, A. (2006). Personality and functional outcome following traumatic brain injury. *Rehabilitation Psychology, 51*, 257–264.

Tomberg, T., Pulver, A., & Tikk, A. (2005). Coping strategies, social support, life orientation and health-related quality of life following traumatic brain injury. *Brain Injury, 19*, 1181–1190.

Waldron-Perrine, B., Rapport, L., Hanks, R., Lumley, M., Meachen, S., & Hubbarth, P. (2011). Religion and spirituality in rehabilitation outcomes among individuals with traumatic brain injury. *Rehabilitation Psychology, 56*(2), 107–116.

World Health Organization, Disability and Rehabilitation Team, United States, Department of Defense & Drucker Brain Injury Center. (2004). *Rehabilitation for persons with traumatic brain injury*. https://apps.who.int/iris/handle/10665/69231

9 Counseling Ambiguous Grief

Case Study

A successful entrepreneur and an experienced triathlete, Thomas was hit by a car as he was training for the bicycle portion of a race. Thomas was married to Evelyn, and together they shared four daughters. This was both of their second marriages. Evelyn came to the marriage with one daughter and Thomas came with twin girls. Together, they had one daughter. When Thomas was injured, he was rushed to the hospital where his family met him. As he lay in a coma, his life and his family's world as they knew it ended. The youngest daughter was still in elementary school, while the other three girls were in college. Coming together to help him recover, every family member took on a different role. Evelyn stayed at the hospital day and night. One daughter took the semester off and came home to care for the youngest daughter and the home. The other two daughters took turns leaving college to help with the family responsibilities.

After Thomas regained consciousness and began rehabilitation, Evelyn was able to go home at night and spend time during the day with her husband. She took a leave of absence from her work as an office manager to help him transition to home and back to normal, or so she thought. Thomas was able to recover from his physical injuries quickly and did not require extended physical rehabilitation. However, he was not the same person. Before the injury, Thomas was laid back, slow to anger, quick humored, organized, and the voice of reason in a house of five women. Once home, it became more obvious that Thomas did not respond in the same way. He could not remember things that he would normally have remembered. He was easily irritated and had a quick temper. Pre-injury, Thomas was comfortable in a loud environment and enjoyed social events with others. Post-injury, Thomas did not want to meet up with his friends or go out of the house. He appeared to get upset if the television was up too loud or on at all. Too many people in the room with too much talking frustrated him. Often, he would leave and seclude himself in his bedroom or office. The family did not know how to respond to him or how to react when he became angry. They also did not understand why he could not remember certain things or why he could not pay attention for extended periods of time. Evelyn and all four daughters began to experience depressive

DOI: 10.4324/9781003301912-9

and anxious symptoms. Eventually, the family began counseling to address the cognitive and emotional deficits and to deal with someone who was not the same person. Evelyn tended to tell Thomas, "You didn't use to lose your temper." Or, "Before, you were my best friend and now I don't know who you are." Thomas would reply with frustration, "I'm not that guy any longer. I can't compete with that guy."

After 18 months, Thomas went back to work. He found that he could not follow normal conversations. He also realized that he was not remembering tasks or details pertinent to a project. He began to use a notebook to put down all his notes and reminders. Thomas worked from home and took naps often when fatigued. After some time, he was able to return to higher functioning but with the memory helps and strategies. The girls all went back to school or college; Evelyn resigned from work and stayed home with her husband. She continued to mourn the loss of the husband she married. She would comment that Thomas was sensitive and kind and even tempered, but now he is so different. She became angry with her family and friends when they would comment that Thomas looks great and seems fine. Outside of a small scar on the side of his head, he did look the same. Unfortunately, he was not the same and their support system could not understand why Evelyn was upset. After several months, Evelyn realized that the old Thomas was gone. She stated that she feels better because she has stopped "looking" for the old person to come back. Their relationship has changed because they both are different. The family of six was joined by a seventh member, brain injury. Although Thomas continues to struggle with his deficits, he has come to appreciate his ability to function and contribute to the family. Evelyn stopped expecting him to be pre-injury Thomas and has enjoyed getting to know the new man and what he can offer to their marriage and their family.

Grief Overview

An acquired or traumatic brain injury creates differences in the physical, emotional, behavioral, and social realms for the individual and the family. Caregivers' roles evolve over the recovery process. The brain injury causes life-changing transitions for the entire family system. Most grief research centers on the reaction to bereavement, whether it is the loss of a loved one, a job, an opportunity, health, or identity. Loss associated with becoming a caretaker for a survivor of brain injury is different from the loss of the loved one through death. The losses are often ongoing and multifaceted, such as adapting to a new everyday life. Pauline Boss, PhD (2010), introduced the term *ambiguous loss*. She defined ambiguous loss as a condition without finality or resolution, which can happen when someone is physically present but psychologically absent. Boss (2006) explained that ambiguous loss "is inherent in the experiences of human migration but also in family life transitions and in unexpected catastrophes of trauma and loss." One client called this kind of loss as emotional losses. She stated that she is unable to travel to see her family, unable to manage her household, unable to cook, unable to return to a career she loved, and unable to be the wife she wanted to be. Thøgersen and Glintborg (2021) studied spouses of survivors of acquired brain injury survivors in Denmark and found that the spouses reported feelings of fear, loneliness, uncertainty, powerlessness, increased responsibility, guilt, and shame. Loneliness was experienced in relation to their partner and in relation to society. The increased responsibility led to increased fatigue, inadequacy, and guilt due to the inability to always meet the expectations of their loved ones. Additionally, the "severity of cognitive impairment in the ABI survivor is associated with the caregiver's experience of ambiguous loss" (Thøgersen & Glintborg, 2021). Common symptoms of the grief felt by survivors are anger, sleep disturbance, depression, despair, fatigue, headaches, distractibility, isolation, withdrawal, and disorganization. A survivor of a cerebrospinal fluid (CSF) leak stated that she misses her former self. While everyone was celebrating her recovery, she felt lonely and grief stricken that she was not the same person as before.

Godwin et al. (2014) found four types of ambiguous loss in relationships after someone experiences a brain injury: (1) loss of you, me, and us; (2) loss of security; (3) loss of connectivity; and (4) loss of future. The loss of you, me, and us was described as the loss of who they have always been and the ways in which that loss has impacted their relationship. The loss of security was described as feeling trapped and insecure at the same time. The insecurities may mean financial challenges or emotional instability. The loss of connectivity means the inability to reach out to the loved one to experience emotional closeness, which can result in loneliness. The loss of future includes the loss of plans, dreams, hopes, and goals that they had as a couple.

The social and cultural influences of grief are important to address. Disenfranchised grief is when a person "experiences a significant loss and their grief is not openly acknowledged, socially validated, or publicly mourned" (Thøgersen & Glintborg, 2021). The lack of social recognition can worsen the reaction to the loss and can add to the confusion of what to call one's own reactions. Psychological and ambiguous loss is associated with disenfranchised grief (Boss, 1999). Loss in connection to living with a disability such as brain injury is not recognized with mourning rituals that are prevalent in the social and cultural world. According to Thøgersen and Glintborg (2021), "social support, combined with social recognition of grief in relation to becoming a caregiver, is essential to the relatives of ABI survivors." Marwit and Kaye (2006) stated that caregiver grief is often "unacknowledged by the majority culture and that some caregivers, as a result, may experience forms of 'complicated grief' that are hard to resolve and that may have serious emotional and even physical consequences." Winslade (1998) suggested that survivors "mourn the loss of those parts of the personality that can't be regained." He recommended that family members "detach themselves from their old expectations and form new ones based on the limited or altered capacities that their son or daughter, brother or sister, spouse or parent now possesses." Landau and Hissett (2008) stated, "While the loss of self, memory, patience, control and confidence are discrepancies that are most severely felt, they are also the most difficult to substantiate, articulate and regain." The survivor of the CSF leak desired for her husband to simply enter the space of her grief whether he understood it or not. His presence was what she wanted.

Identity Changes

Both caregivers and survivors of brain injury expressed the need to identify who they are now as opposed to who they were pre-injury. Godwin et al. (2014) found that survivors described their transformation of personal identity as the death of the former self and the re-emergence of a new self. The loss of self that they attribute to their new physical and emotional deficits significantly altered their relationships with family and friends. According to Nochi (1998), there are "three categories of loss of self: loss of clear self-knowledge, loss of self by comparison, and loss of self in the eyes of others" (Landau & Hissett, 2008). Having a diminished role in the family system is particularly difficult. For example, not being the breadwinner of the family or not being able to complete common everyday tasks can make the survivor distraught and troubled because s/he cannot meet his/her own expectations or the expectations of others. For example, one primary caregiver mentioned that she saw herself more as a parent than a spouse. She stated that it was easier for her to think of her husband as a child, not just as her husband.

A coping strategy is to renegotiate personal and family boundaries. Landau and Hissett (2008) found that survivors of mTBI felt a disconnect between who they present to the world and who they feel they have become inside. They also reported shutting down emotionally, which created confusion among family members as to how to react or respond. When a loved one first sustains a brain injury, there is no boundary ambiguity because the family members take on extra roles. It is when the rehabilitation process does not conform to the preconceived timeline that "tolerance was reduced, impatience grew, tempers became frayed, and relationships at best were strained," leading to boundary ambiguity (Landau & Hissett, 2008).

Ambiguous loss is considered to be the most stressful kind of loss because it defies closure (Landau & Hissett, 2008). Families who contained a member with a brain injury appeared to "struggle with the realization that the injury has left a stranger in their midst who has become the predominant presence in every conversation and major decision." As mentioned earlier, when there is the death of a family member, "it is validated through the sociocultural processes that allow families to move forward through their grief" (Landau & Hissett, 2008). However, when a family member experiences a brain injury and the family is not acknowledged by social processes, it can create a boundary ambiguity within the family system. This can paralyze the family, making it difficult for them to grieve and heal. Boundary ambiguity "may manifest as loss of the injured person as the family knew him or her, as well as loss of the family system as it once was" (Landau & Hissett, 2008). The mom of a TBI survivor said that she did not think she would ever forget it or get over it because, "I look at her and just think how she used to be. But she's good now, but I remember before" (personal communication, January 20, 2012).

After an injury, couples strive to re-establish their previous relationship but soon realize that the striving to become who they used to be is futile. Instead, couples can learn to establish new rituals, create a new relationship, and envision a new future (Godwin et al., 2014). The new relationship consists of creating new roles and responsibilities for everyday existence. One couple in counseling shared their experience. Josh was injured when the tractor he was driving overturned. He suffered a severe traumatic brain injury and was in a coma for two weeks. As the main breadwinner of the family, he was unable to continue full-time work and eventually had to retire. His wife, Rachel, went to work full time to supplement their income. Although the role change was difficult for both of them, they acclimated by seeing their new responsibilities as a new way to love one another. Rachel said that her husband is different. He is not the same person as he was before the injury. During a couple's session (personal communication, March 8, 2021), she said, "I just tell people that I've been married to two men but didn't have to get a divorce!" They had family and social support to help them navigate the ambiguous losses associated with his injury. However, according to Josh and Rachel, they had to educate their friends, church, and family. Godwin et al. (2014) found that couples who maintained their marriage or relationship post-injury had intentional purpose, regenerated connection, developed a tolerance of ambiguity, and refined commitment.

Counseling Considerations

It is essential for a counselor to recognize the possibility of ambiguous loss and boundary ambiguity when working with a family who has a member with a brain injury. Involving the family system in the counseling process as soon as possible helps to mitigate the results of ambiguous grief. It is helpful to allow the family to discuss their feelings of fear, guilt, shame, anger, or helplessness as a means of giving them a safe outlet. Additionally, educating them about what is a normal reaction to an abnormal event normalizes their reactions without the accompanying feelings of guilt or shame. Learning to accept the differences caused by the brain injury within their family system and their personal relationships can be comforting and reassuring. A great example of this comes from the wife of a survivor of TBI who said that she cannot blame her husband for what happened to him because it was not his fault. She stated that she could not compare him to his old self because she could not force him to live in the shadow of someone he is not.

Boundary ambiguity is worsened when families are unable to communicate about the painful topics and resort to secrecy. Clear communication about their observations of the loss and changes in the individual can be restorative. At this point, they can work together to develop compensatory strategies to further navigate the deficits, while creating space to improve. When survivors understand their problems, they can take an active role in their own recovery. A family therapist can work within the family system to regenerate confidence, reconstruct identity, build tolerance for ambiguity, identify resources, and foster support and acceptance (Landau & Hissett, 2008).

It would be remiss for a counselor to direct the family to simply concentrate on the losses and not shift their perspective to the gains that have been acquired since the injury. Not only does this convey hope, but it also offers the opportunity to appreciate the strengths that have come from the difficulties. Ruff and Chester (2014) recommend giving equal diligence to strengths in the emotional, cognitive, spiritual, physical, and social realms. They further explain that deficits are not the same as disabilities. Deficits include "impairments that allow the individual to continue to function as before but perhaps at a reduced level of efficiency or with accommodations." Deficits tend to change over time and often interact with one another. As the person heals, some deficits become less pronounced. On the other hand, disability "will not improve and prevents an individual from continuing to function effectively as he or she had previously done educationally, vocationally, and/or psychosocially" (Ruff & Chester, 2014).

There are two counseling theories that address the issue of ambiguous loss. The Adlerian concept of compensation addresses the need to compensate for losses and to preserve personal integrity and independence. For brain injury, compensatory strategies are more than coping skills. They are the process of creating new ways of accomplishing the same goal. Narrative psychology offers the survivor the opportunity to create a self-narrative of how s/he relates to the world post-injury. One client stated that she accepts that she is different post-TBI and has different abilities. She stated that she focuses not on what she has lost but on the things she can do now. She is re-creating her life to accommodate her injury, and she volunteers at her state brain injury association.

Christian Counseling

Clients have found certain biblical references and spiritual beliefs helpful in dealing with ambiguous grief. For example, Romans 8:28 (New Living Translation, NLT) "And we know that God causes everything to work together for the good of those who love God and are called according to his purpose for them." This is not to say that all things are good or that suffering is good. It says that God creates something good out of the suffering. Patti Foster, the survivor of TBI mentioned earlier in the book, stated that God redeemed her pain with a whole new purpose and passion for helping those around the world who have a brain injury. A client shared that she tries to take hold of every opportunity that God has given her since the injury. She admits that she vents to God about her feelings, which she finds very helpful.

In response to the unwelcome reality of ambiguous loss, the Apostle Paul discussed another spiritual truth that could be applied. Second Corinthians 5:17 (NASB) states, "Therefore if anyone is in Christ, he is a new creature; the old things passed away; behold new things have come." In the Old Testament, a promise from God in Isaiah 43:19 (NIV) states, "See, I am doing a new thing! Now it springs up; do you not perceive it? I am making a way in the desert and streams in the wasteland." Embracing the new self and recognizing that God was making a way in what appeared to be barrenness can comfort those struggling with the deficits of TBI. Faith in God's promise of renewal appears to offer hope for survivors and families learning how to navigate the new life created by the devastation of TBI. The truth that God's call on one's life does not change is also helpful. It may expand or narrow, but the call is the same. Romans 11:29 (NIV) says, "for God's gifts and his call are irrevocable." Rick suffered a TBI from a motor vehicle accident. He had two passions before the injury, preaching and football. Since his injury, Rick has been sharing the Gospel as he participates in physical rehabilitation and recovery and through various speaking engagements. He stated that he still wants to be a full-time evangelist, but he got started sharing his testimony with other survivors and the therapists who are helping him recover. His desire to share God with others never changed.

As a Christian counselor, reminding clients of the character of God as they experience loss can be comforting. Share truths such as God is with them in the pain, just as He was with them in the peace. For example, in Deuteronomy 31:6 (NIV), He says, "Be strong and courageous. Do not be afraid . . . for the Lord your God goes with you; he will never leave you nor forsake you." During traumatic times, it can be normal not to feel God's presence. But He is there whether He is "felt" or not. God does not act in opposition to His character. Therefore, He will bring benefit out of pain. God says that "you will experience [his] peace, which exceeds anything we can understand." (Philippians 4:7 NLT). Often, clients say that they did not worry about whether they would live. There was a peace that they could not explain knowing that everything would be all right. One client who suffered a brain injury from a blast stated that she would not change anything because the injury brought her closer to God. Another belief that survivors have found helpful is that their brain has been injured, but their spirit has not. Their connection with God has not been injured. Clients have shared that knowing this has helped them transition from thinking only of their losses to concentrating on what they gained or did not lose.

Faith Alternatives

For people of all faiths and non-faiths, identity reconstruction was recommended by Landau and Hissett (2008). Part of this process is reframing the perceived loss as a blessing in disguise. Reports of a greater appreciation of life, greater compassion, and a newly formed dedication to holistic health were outcomes mentioned in their study. According to Landau and Hissett (2008), the survivors of mTBI that they studied stated that identity reconstruction was made possible if "they were given time to heal, were able to sleep restfully, learned to set reasonable goals, and made specific time for relaxation and leisure with their partners and family members." One client stated that he misses what he used to be able to do, but he tries to get busy with what he can do.

Meditation is an effective means of processing loss. There are different types of meditation depending on one's beliefs or moral tenets. For example, meditations such as chakra, guided imagery, Vipassana, metta Buddhist, and transcendental guide one through the feelings of loss to a sense of peace and awareness. Chakra meditation helps one to identify the energy center in the body that may block grief. The goal is to meet the losses with the awareness and wisdom already in the body, mind, and spirit, thereby manifesting a new state of balance. Guided imagery concentrates on the concept that, with every goodbye, there is also a connection. There are several scripts available that take one through various images that provide an experience of emotion associated with loss and develop a deeper sense of love and appreciation of the losses. Vipassana meditation, also considered insight meditation, helps one to see things as they really are and to recognize the whole from the self. Metta or Buddhist meditation encourages one to practice loving kindness and comfort when grieving. Transcendental meditation incorporates a mantra that is repeated for several minutes each day. The goal is to restore calm and relaxation, process grief, and continue the task of living.

Because ambiguous grief is closely associated with the lack of acknowledgment from society and culture, it is imperative that the client's local church body (temple, parish, synagogue, etc.) be educated on how to help the family deal with losses associated with brain injury. A part of the recognition and acknowledgment of the loss may include setting aside a time to mourn the ambiguous losses within a personal and community setting. When counseling a survivor of brain injury or his/her family member, it is helpful to explain the process of grief that honors the lost part of the person or identity or role or whatever the loss may be. The part that was lost is important. It served a purpose and functioned to bring quality to the person's life. Therefore, it is important to put that "part" in a place of honor in one's mind. As opposed to burying and forgetting something, dedicate the old self to a special place that is respected and safe. Sometimes clients may picture a special container in their mind where their old self is located. Others decide to have an actual picture or representation of themselves to see and appreciate.

Stoler and Hill (1998) suggested steps to heal the loss of self and other losses associated with brain injury. The first step is to acknowledge the reality of the loss and to acknowledge that brain injury has made one a new person. The second step is to identify and express grief. The third step is to communicate the losses by collecting mementos of one's former self. The fourth step is to acknowledge the ambivalence of surviving a brain injury, both the positive and negative feelings about living, and to put the feelings in the perspective of the new self. The fifth step is to learn to let it go by moving forward with one's life. The final step is to move on with the understanding that one must relinquish the plans and dreams of the former self and rethink one's goals on the basis of present strengths and abilities.

Conclusion

The role of ambiguous grief within the family affected by brain injury is not as well studied as grief associated with death. Pauline Boss, PhD, coined the term ambiguous loss to describe when someone is physically present but psychologically absent. This chapter gave an overview of the grieving issues associated with brain injury, which include boundary ambiguity, identity changes, and role reversals. Counseling considerations from Alfred Adler and from narrative psychology were also discussed, along with biblical references for those of the Christian faith. Various meditations were presented from different faith groups that address loss and peace. The next chapter addresses posttraumatic stress disorder and its variants regarding brain injury.

References

Boss, P. (1999). *Ambiguous loss*. Harvard University Press.

Boss, P. (2006). *Loss, trauma, and resilience: Therapeutic work with ambiguous loss*. W.W. Norton & Company.

Boss, P. (2010). The trauma and complicated grief of ambiguous loss. *Pastoral Psychology, 59*, 137–145.

Godwin, E., Chappell, B., & Kreutzer, J. (2014). Relationships after TBI: A grounded research study. *Brain Injury, 28*(4), 398–413. https://doi.org/10.3109/02699052.2014.880514

Landau, J., & Hissett, J. (2008). Mild traumatic brain injury: Impact on identity and ambiguous loss in the family. *Families, Systems, & Health, 26*(1), 69–85. https://doi.org/10.1037/1091-7527.26.1.69

Marwit, S., & Kaye, P. (2006). Measuring grief in caregivers of persons with acquired brain injury. *Brain Injury, 20*(13–14), 1419–1429. https://doi.org/10.1080/02699050601082214

Nochi, M. (1998). "Loss of self" in the narratives of people with traumatic brain injuries: A qualitative analysis. *Social Science & Medicine, 46*, 869–878.

Ruff, R., & Chester, S. (2014). *Effective psychotherapy for individuals with brain injury*. Guilford Press.

Stoler, D., & Hill, B. (1998). *Coping with mild traumatic brain injury: A guide to living with the challenges associated with concussion/brain injury*. Avery.

Thøgersen, C., & Glintborg, C. (2021). Ambiguous loss and disenfranchised grief among spouses of brain injury survivors. *Nordic Psychology, 74*(1), 16–29. https://doi.org/10.1080/19012276.2020.1862699

Winslade, W. (1998). *Confronting traumatic brain injury: Devastation, hope, and healing*. Yale University Press.

10 Counseling Posttraumatic Stress

Case Study

At age 45, Josh had a successful medical career, was married with a wonderful family of two daughters, and had a myriad of friends. During a weekend getaway, Josh was riding in a boat with two of his friends and their daughters when suddenly their boat slammed into a cement bridge. It was late at night and there were no reflectors on the bridge. One of his friends sitting at the front of the boat was struck by the bridge and died instantly. Josh's head hit the bridge as well, causing a severe TBI. His teenage daughter, Abby, called the paramedics. His family and friends gathered at the emergency department waiting for news about whether Josh would survive his injuries. His life hung in the balance as his family sat dazed, wondering what had happened. After three weeks in acute care, he was transferred to transitional rehabilitation where he spent several months. Abby was in high school at the time, and she later stated that she could not talk about what happened with anyone except her mom and sister. Even after months of rehabilitation, Josh was unable to maintain his medical practice and sold it to another physician. He continued various outpatient therapies over the course of the next year. Because of the catastrophic nature of the accident, litigation was pursued by Josh and his family, which added another level of stress to the family. Although he did not remember the actual accident, Josh did recall certain details of his recovery and eventually was told that his friend was killed in the boat wreck. Post-accident treatment, litigation, loss of his business, family trauma, and the inability to perform at the high level he was able to pre-injury all contributed to Josh experiencing posttraumatic stress disorder. His daughter Abby did not experience a brain injury, but she did remember all of the incident, including her dad falling into her arms unconscious and bleeding profusely. Josh's older daughter was away at college when the accident happened. She came home to be with the family for a short time. Josh and Abby began counseling separately. Abby also participated in art therapy, which she found helpful. For several years, Abby was unable to relate to people her age and felt as though no one could really understand all that she had experienced. She also felt "stuck" at the age of the accident. Abby suffered from flashbacks, hypervigilance, helplessness, hopelessness, and feeling detached

DOI: 10.4324/9781003301912-10

from others. Josh struggled with losing his livelihood and practice, not trusting his brain, not understanding how it was injured, and what happened to his friend who died. He also suffered from feelings of abandonment, helplessness, and hopelessness and avoided the lake and boat. He also suffered PTSD from all of the legal proceedings that required him to seek additional medical help and to participate in mediation and depositions. His wife, a stay-at-home mom, was forced to take on all of the household and financial responsibilities, which in the end became too much for her.

After several years, the litigation was resolved, the rehabilitation services ended, and Josh recovered well enough to consider returning to medicine. He believes that he may be able to practice on a limited basis. Abby graduated from high school, entered university, and hopes to become an art therapist. Unfortunately, Josh's wife decided to divorce him. Their other daughter went on to get her doctorate in theatrical studies.

Overview

Posttraumatic stress disorder (PTSD) symptoms were first recognized during the American Civil War in the 1860s. At that time, posttraumatic symptoms were associated with cardiovascular disease by Dr. Jacob Mendes Da Costa, who coined the term "soldier's heart" also known as Da Costa syndrome. During World War I, a similar characterization of the soldiers returning from battle was called "shell shock." Psychological theories proposed that the same phenomenon followed the constructs of nostalgia, war neurosis, combat fatigue, and combat exhaustion (Monson et al., 2007). In 1941, psychiatrist Abram Kardiner stated that the psychological and physiological responses to combat could be characterized as physioneurosis. While working at a local veteran's hospital, he identified that his patients were triggered by sensory stimuli, causing them to experience panic attacks and flashbacks to their combat experience. Kardiner's work became the foundation of studies of combat-related trauma. Posttraumatic stress disorder became a diagnosable condition in 1980 when it appeared in the third edition of the *Diagnostic and Statistical Manual of Mental Disorders* published by the American Psychiatric Association.

PTSD is considered one of the Trauma- and Stressor-Related Disorders in the *Diagnostic and Statistical Manual of Mental Disorders, Fifth Edition* (DSM-V). To be diagnosed with PTSD, one must have been exposed to actual or threatened death, serious injury, or sexual violence by either directly experiencing the trauma, witnessing the trauma, learning that a trauma happened to a close friend or family member, or experiencing repeated exposure to aversive details of the trauma event. Additionally, the person experiences a combination of the following: recurrent or intrusive memories, distressing dreams, flashbacks, aversive reactions to triggering events, avoidance of stimuli associated with the trauma, inability to remember an important aspect of the trauma, irritability, hypervigilance, exaggerated startle response, self-destructive behavior, feeling detached or a negative emotional state, inability to experience positive emotions, or sleep disturbance (APA, 2013). The latest criteria for PTSD removed the "subjective experience of fear, helplessness and horror during or after the trauma, include[d] a new cluster of alterations in cognition/mood and added three symptoms including negative emotional states, blame/guilt, and reckless behaviour" (Tanev et al., 2014).

Some believe that their brain injury worked in their favor during a traumatic event. Rosa Blum, a survivor of the Holocaust (personal communication, January 3, 2021), stated that the brain injury she experienced from an assault by Josef Mengele was protective for her. She stated that the brain injury kept her from fully comprehending the atrocities she experienced in Auschwitz. Although she experienced multiple traumatic events, their full magnitude was beyond her ability to understand.

The prevalence of PTSD after TBI varies from 3% to 59% (Gill et al., 2014). Part of the issue is that some of the symptoms of the two overlap, making it difficult to discern between them. Over the past couple of decades, some studies have suggested that PTSD and TBI do not and could not coexist. They are considered to be mutually incompatible disorders because people who suffer PTSD cannot forget the traumatic event and those who suffer a TBI cannot remember the event. However, recent studies have suggested that "organic amnesia associated with TBI (post-traumatic amnesia (PTA) and retrograde amnesia (RA)) might offer little or no protection against developing PTSD" (King, 2008).

Recently reported incidence rates of PTSD for survivors of TBI are equal to or greater than the rates for those who have not suffered a brain injury. Al-Ozairi et al. (2015) found that survivors of brain injury across the severity spectrum (mild, moderate, and severe) experience symptoms of PTSD "notwithstanding the participants' inability to remember the nature of the trauma experienced." They continued: "[T]he participants who appear most vulnerable to the development of intrusive and avoidant symptoms are those whose memories start returning on a consistent basis within an hour of injury." This suggests that the survivor will remember the immediate post-accident sequence of events, such as extraction from a vehicle, the chaos of an accident scene, the emergency department procedures, and the uncertainty and fear surrounding one or more of the experiences.

King (2008) stated that there are four mechanisms whereby someone with a TBI may experience PTSD. The first mechanism is if the person experiences a mild TBI and there is no memory loss. The second mechanism is when the person has pockets of memory although is amnesic for other segments of the trauma. The third mechanism occurs when there is no explicit memory, but the trauma is re-experienced by an unconscious or implicit fear response. The fourth mechanism also occurs when there is no explicit memory, but the survivor has been given information about the event or s/he has imagined what happened and thereby constructed pseudo memories. Of course, the aftermath of the trauma may cause PTSD, such as painful medical procedures or frightening experiences or perceptions when the person emerges from a coma.

Vasterling et al. (2019) addressed the reason why there may be PTSD with TBI. Factors that contribute to the dual diagnosis include

> implicit (unconscious) encoding of affective and sensory experiences (e.g., sights and smells) associated with the traumatic event, conscious encoding of some aspects of the event, reconstruction of the trauma memory from secondary sources (e.g., family, other observers), and memory of circumstances surrounding the event that also may be psychologically traumatic (e.g., sights at the scene of an accident after consciousness was regained).

The coexistence of TBI and PTSD is further explained by the dual-representation theory, which states "that some degree of consciousness is essential for the creation of any kind of trauma memory" (Harvey et al., 2005).

Overlapping Symptomology

As mentioned earlier, the symptoms of PTSD and TBI overlap, especially in mild traumatic brain injury. A thorough assessment of the symptoms and their origin is imperative in diagnosing the client. During the initial session, addressing issues that are specific to PTSD such as hyperalertness, flashbacks, nightmares, re-experience of the trauma, or avoidance of trigger events, people, or situations will help to differentiate the diagnosis. It is helpful to also ask questions addressing specific TBI symptomology, such as headaches, nausea, cognitive fatigue, balance problems, dizziness, and disorganized thoughts. Their common symptoms are concentration difficulties, memory problems, irritability, anxiety, and sleep disturbance.

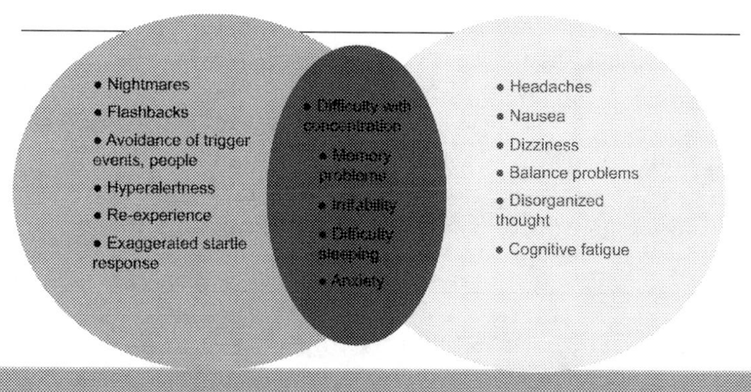

Figure 10.1 Symptoms of PTSD and mTBI.

PTSD and mTBI

There are also significant differences in the symptomology of PTSD and mTBI. For example, the poor emotional expression in PTSD "represents emotional blunting rather than [the] apathy (or lack of initiation) of traumatic brain injury" (Coetzer, 2010). The memory loss associated with PTSD is not the same as the forgetting of everyday events or the difficulty with new learning that accompanies TBI. Coetzer (2010) further explained that "sleep disturbances in post traumatic stress disorder tend to be in response to anxiety, rumination, and nightmares, whereas in traumatic brain injury there can be hypersomnia or hyposomnia, sometimes related to pain or other biological factors."

Counseling Considerations

According to King (2008), the current literature suggests that there "are no PTSD treatments specifically designed for patients with the dual diagnosis with a robust evidence base." The literature suggests that cognitive-behavioral therapy (CBT) may be effective because it is a recommended technique for PTSD in the general population. Utilization of adaptive forms of CBT appears to address the cognitive impairment and post-concussive symptoms. King (2002) cautioned against exposure therapy whereby the client recounts the traumatic experience, because "such interventions could precipitate traumatic perseveration." Perseveration occurs when there are lesions in the frontal, occipital, and parietal areas of the brain. It is a "form of cognitive and behavioural inflexibility which causes difficulties in altering an existing response once environmental demands do not require the response any longer" (King, 2002). King (2002) recommended techniques to help alleviate the prospect of perseveration. These recommendations create a safety net for the client as s/he discusses the trauma. Nonexposure aspects of treatment should be addressed before exposure-based work is tackled. Grounding skills (focusing on the five senses in the environment) and distraction should be introduced as means of reducing heightened emotional and cognitive responses.

Cognitive rehabilitation has been shown to be an effective treatment for brain injury. Evidence supports "attention training (graded exercises to stimulate attention) and metacognitive strategies (feedback, self-monitoring, self-regulation, strategy use) that promote generalization of the cognitive rehabilitation to real world tasks" (Tanev et al., 2014). However, there have been limited studies supporting the effectiveness of cognitive rehabilitation to treat PTSD.

Non-Faith- or Faith-Based Counseling

For those who do not prescribe to a specific faith, the following are treatment options. Psychoeducation is an important component to treating PTSD for a survivor of brain injury. A description of the symptoms of PTSD, how to manage them, and what the progression of recovery looks like are part of the psychoeducation. Trauma-focused treatment such as eye movement desensitization and reprocessing is a newer approach that has not been fully studied regarding its efficacy for survivors of brain injury. Cognitive-behavioral therapy helps with the reduction of symptoms of PTSD. Acceptance and Commitment Therapy has been introduced as an approach to help with the co-morbidity.

Eye Movement Desensitization and Reprocessing

In 1989, Francine Shapiro developed eye movement desensitization and reprocessing (EMDR), a technique that utilizes eye movement for cognitive restructuring of traumatic memories. The client chooses the traumatic material on which to focus. The clinician uses an instrument that the client follows across his/her visual field as s/he concentrates on past trauma. The client identifies more positive or adaptive thoughts with the trauma memory. The exercise activates the acceleration of information processing, which is the product of "dual attention to present stimuli and past trauma, a differential effect of 'neuronal bursts' caused by the various repetitive movements or deconditioning caused by a relaxation response" (Monson et al., 2007). Research on the effectiveness of EMDR for brain injury is varied. It is considered a variant of cognitive-behavioral therapy and trauma-focused therapy. I would suggest that this technique be utilized after the client cognitively recovers well enough to fully benefit from it.

Cognitive-Behavioral Therapy

Although there is no gold standard for treating PTSD and TBI, adaptations of cognitive-behavioral therapy (CBT) have been recommended. Ponsford (2013) stated that CBT may reduce some of the symptoms of PTSD and negative emotions. CBT incorporates psychoeducation, anxiety management, and cognitive restructuring. The psychoeducation portion of CBT "provides information about common symptoms following a traumatic event, normalizes the trauma reactions, and establishes a rationale for treatment" (Bryant & Litz, 2012). Anxiety management includes relaxation techniques, deep breathing, and self-talk. Cognitive restructuring helps clients to reconstruct negative automatic thoughts into an adaptive, effective, positive means of interpreting their beliefs about the trauma, the self, and the world.

Acceptance and Commitment Therapy

Acceptance and Commitment Therapy (ACT) was developed by Steven Hayes, PhD in 1999, to help clients to identify and work toward goals. The technique employs mindfulness and behavioral change processes to create a meaningful life, while accepting the pain that inevitably accompanies it (Hayes et al., 2013). ACT does not attempt to directly stop negative emotions but rather encourages individuals to develop a compassionate relationship with them. The model values improved quality of life rather than symptom reduction and allows for the deficits associated with brain injury.

Christian Counseling

Counseling from a biblical perspective requires an understanding of how the subject of trauma is addressed within the holy scriptures. In Greek, "trauma" means "wound" and is located only in Luke 10:34 (NAS), in which the good Samaritan approaches the person who had been beaten and robbed. He "came to him and bandaged up his wounds, pouring oil and wine on them; and he put him on his beast, and brought him to an inn and took care of him." The concepts of woundedness and suffering, however, are addressed extensively throughout the Bible.

The question of where God is in suffering is the basic tenet of theodicy. Although most clients will not enter a counselor's office asking about the intricacies of theodicy, they will ask why God lets suffering happen. Or, where is God in the middle of chaos? In counseling, I find it helpful to refer to Genesis 1:2 (NIV), which says, "Now the earth was formless and empty, darkness was over the surface of the deep, and the Spirit of God was hovering over the waters." When someone is traumatized and suffers a brain injury, his/her world becomes formless and empty. It may feel like chaos and seem dark with no shape or purpose. Often families do not know what to do or where to turn. As faith-based counselors, we introduce them to the truth that God has been there all along. The Spirit of God hovered over the accident scene, the diagnosis, and the treatment. He brought "good Samaritans" in the form of physiatrists, neurologists, nurses, and therapists to bind the wounds and take care of their loved one. The "inn" is the hospital, the rehabilitation facility, and the consistent, around-the-clock care needed for healing.

Another aspect of brain injury is the tension between suffering, comfort, and hope. Isaiah 43:19 (NET) states, "Look, I am about to do something new. Now it begins to happen! Do you not recognize it? Yes, I will make a road in the wilderness and paths in the wastelands." Patti Foster (personal communication, March 31, 2022) interprets that scripture as follows:

> [D]on't try to make yourself the same person you were before the brain injury. Do your best with what you have, on the other side of the injury, and make the most of every adjustment brain injury has made of you – embrace it and let it shine life and hope that has [*sic*] purpose!

She further explains that when

> learning to live again after the injury, we don't need to base our after-injury lives on our former life nor dwell on the things of our past life, but accept, lean into, and embrace the edits and adjustments of our new life after the

> injury. Brain injury usually happens out of the box, so we usually need to meet it in ways that are out of the box.

The Bible connects meaning and hope during suffering. Psalm 23:4 (NIV) reminds the reader, "Even though I walk through the darkest valley, I will fear no evil, for you are with me; your rod and your staff, they comfort me." Several survivors of brain injury who have leaned on their faith share the verses that helped them. Rebecca, who experienced a brain injury and a brain tumor, took comfort in Romans 8:18 (NKJV): "For I consider that the sufferings of this present time are not worthy to be compared with the glory which shall be revealed in us." Denise, a caregiver, stated that she daily read 2 Corinthians 1:3–4 (NIV):

> Praise be to the God and Father of our Lord Jesus Christ, the Father of compassion and the God of all comfort, who comforts us in all our troubles, so that we can comfort those in any trouble with the comfort we ourselves receive from God.

Marcy, the caregiver for her husband who suffered a brain injury by falling off the roof, stated that Philippians 4:4–7 (NIV) helped her:

> Rejoice in the Lord always. I will say it again: Rejoice! Let your gentleness be evident to all. The Lord is near. Do not be anxious about anything, but in every situation, by prayer and petition, with thanksgiving, present your requests to God. And the peace of God, which transcends all understanding, will guard your hearts and your minds in Christ Jesus.

Patti, whose story is shared in Chapter 3, stated that Psalm 40:1–3 (NIV) became her foundational verse.

> I waited patiently for the Lord; he inclined to me and heard my cry. He drew me up from the desolate pit, out of the miry bog, and set my feet upon a rock, making my steps secure. He put a new song in my mouth, a song of praise to our God. Many will see and fear, and put their trust in the Lord.

These scriptures combine one's present suffering with the belief, hope, and trust that God is present and will do what He promises.

A reframing of the traumatic experience considering Genesis 50:20 (NIV) – "You intended to harm me, but God intended it for good to accomplish what is now being done, the saving of many lives" – establishes a bigger perspective and greater purpose through suffering. When working with survivors of brain injury who exhibit PTSD symptoms, it is important to ask how they see or perceive the harm done to them considering their understanding of God and His plan for their future. Most survivors want to contribute to the lives of others by sharing what they have learned through their experience. Many have mentioned that giving back by sharing with others helps them to see and experience a greater purpose. It embodies hope in the midst of and despite their suffering.

The example of Christ himself who suffered trauma on the cross (including a crown of thorns pushed into his head) demonstrates the redemptive quality of trauma. It was his wounds, his scars that bring healing to those who also suffer. The disciple Thomas stated that he would not believe that Christ died and rose from the dead "unless I see the nail marks in his hands and put my finger where the nails were, and put my hand into his side, I will not believe." (John 20:25, NIV). Thomas' resistance was met with Jesus' grace. He appeared to Thomas and said in John 20:27 (NIV), "Put your finger here; see my hands. Reach out your hand and put it in my side. Stop doubting and believe." Jesus gave survivors an example of the redemptive aspect of sharing personal scars with one another. When a survivor can tell another survivor his/her story, the listener begins to feel heard, understood, and not alone. Allowing one's personal scars to bring hope and comfort to others enriches the lives of survivors and establishes an ongoing opportunity to create purpose through the suffering.

Conclusion

This chapter focused on the prevalence of posttraumatic stress within the brain injury population. There remains an ongoing debate as to whether a survivor of TBI can also experience PTSD. Different parts of the debate were described, along with the complications of diagnosing each problem due to the overlap of symptoms such as sleep disturbance, memory issues, and concentration problems. At the time of this writing, treatment modalities to address PTSD in individuals with TBI have been developed, although research is needed to document the efficacy of each. Cognitive-behavioral therapy, EMDR, ACT, and psychoeducation are a few of the recommended therapeutic methods. Last, for faith-based counselors, there are a plethora of verses in the Old Testament and New Testament acknowledging the existence of trauma and offering truths of God's plan and hope in spite of and in the midst of suffering. Several survivors of brain injury and their caregivers shared their favorite verses that bring them comfort and direction in response to the trauma of brain injury. The next chapter focuses on the anger and fatigue experienced by survivors of brain injury. Practical strategies and counseling techniques to alleviate the effects of anger and fatigue after a brain injury are addressed.

References

Al-Ozairi, A., McCullagh, S., & Feinstein, A. (2015). Predicting posttraumatic stress symptoms following mild, moderate, and severe traumatic brain injury: The role of posttraumatic amnesia. *Journal of Head Trauma Rehabilitation, 30*(4), 283–289.

American Psychiatric Association. (2013). *Diagnostic and statistical manual of mental disorders* (5th ed.).

Bryant, R., & Litz, B. (2012). Treatment of posttraumatic stress disorder following mild traumatic brain injury. In J. Vasterling, R. Bryant, & T. Keane (Eds.), *PTSD and mild traumatic brain injury* (pp. 219–234). Guilford Press.

Coetzer, R. (2010). *Anxiety and mood disorders following traumatic brain injury: Clinical assessment and psychotherapy*. Routledge Press.

Gill, I., Mullin, S., & Simpson, J. (2014). Psychosocial and psychological factors associated with post-traumatic stress disorder following traumatic brain injury in adult civilian populations: A systematic review. *Brain Injury, 28*(1), 1–14. https://doi.org/10.3109/02699052.2013.851416

Harvey, A., Kopelman, M., & Brewin, C. (2005). PTSD and traumatic brain injury. In J. Vasterling & C. Brewin (Eds.), *Neuropsychology of PTSD: Biological, cognitive, and clinical perspectives* (pp. 230–246). Guilford Press.

Hayes, S., Levin, M., Plumb-Vilardaga, J., Villatte, J., & Pistorello, J. (2013). Acceptance and commitment therapy and contextual behavioral science: Examining the progress of a distinctive model of behavioral and cognitive therapy. *Behavior Therapy, 44*(2), 180–198.

King, N. (2002). Perseveration of traumatic re-experiencing in PTSD; a cautionary note regarding exposure based psychological treatments for PTSD when head injury and dysexecutive impairment are also present. *Brain Injury, 16*(1), 65–74. https://doi.org/10.1080/02699050110088263

King, N. (2008). PTSD and traumatic brain injury: Folklore and fact? *Brain Injury, 22*(1), 1–5. https://doi.org/10.1080/02699050701829696

Monson, C., Friedman, M., & La Bash, H. (2007). A psychological history of PTSD. In M. Friedman, T. Keane, & P. Resick (Eds.), *Handbook of PTSD: Science and practice* (pp. 37–52). Guilford Press.

Ponsford, J. (2013). Dealing with the impact of TBI on psychological adjustment and relationships. In J. Ponsford, S. Sloan, & P. Snow (Eds.), *Traumatic brain injury: Rehabilitation for everyday adaptive living* (2nd ed., pp. 226–262). Psychology Press.

Tanev, K., Pentel, K., Kredlow, M., & Charney, M. (2014). PTSD and TBI co-morbidity: Scope, clinical presentation and treatment options. *Brain Injury, 28*(3), 261–270. https://doi.org/10.3109/02699052.2013.873821

Vasterling, J., Jacob, S., & Rasmusson, A. (2019). Posttraumatic stress disorder. In J. Silver, T. McAllister, & D. Arciniegas (Eds.), *Textbook of traumatic brain injury* (3rd ed., pp. 361–378). American Psychiatric Association Publishing.

11 Counseling Fatigue and Anger

Case Study

Rick was traveling back from a high school football game when he was struck head-on by another vehicle. He has no memory of the wreck or what caused it. All he knew was that he was in the hospital with his family all around his bed. Rick had great hopes for his future. He was going to sign to play football at an out-of-state university the day after his wreck. He wanted to preach the Gospel after college. Neither of those goals was in his near future, if at all. As he was a "nice Christian young man," his family was surprised to hear the words coming out of his mouth in the hospital! No one had heard him use profanity for as long as they had known him. They did not understand what changed. As he was discharged from the acute hospital and transitioned to the rehabilitation facility, his language and temper did not improve. His family blamed themselves. They blamed the treatment team. They wanted him to have medication to help. They scolded him for his loss of self-control. Fortunately, one of the physical medicine and rehabilitation physicians explained to them that Rick's brain was angry, not Rick. This is common with traumatic brain injury. In fact, it is a sign that he is recovering, the doctor said. The nursing staff and therapists encouraged the family to ignore the profanity and walk out of the room if Rick loses his temper. When he is appropriate, encourage him and remain positive. "Sometimes it is helpful to change the subject," they recommended.

Fatigue was another noticeable difference in Rick. Before the wreck, he was a go-getter . . . always doing something. He would go to school, go to practice, hang out with friends, go home, and do homework. Now, he could barely manage a brief therapy session without needing to nap for one to two hours. It seemed that the smallest tasks wore him out. To carry on a conversation for more than a couple of minutes was too much for him. And when he was fatigued, his angry outbursts were more frequent. The treatment team recommended that Rick have only one guest at a time. Anyone in his room was to only speak about positive topics. His family were also encouraged to slow down and not talk too fast or move too fast. The reduction in sensory stimulation and therapy responsibilities helped Rick to calm down. Eventually, he was able to recognize when he was fatigued and irritable. His family asked him to

DOI: 10.4324/9781003301912-11

share when he was at his limit, and they would leave him alone. Quiet and rest seemed to help the most.

Years after his injury, Rick still occasionally deals with anger and irritation, mostly when there is too much activity around him or when too much is being asked of him. He continues in outpatient physical and speech therapies. To his family's delight, he has decided to try to go back to the ministry. He prays for God to help him control his tongue and to be kind to himself and rest when he is fatigued. Rick practices gratitude to his family and friends. He believes that he is a miracle and is hopeful of sharing his story with people all over the world.

Overview

Fatigue and anger are two of the most common symptoms of brain injury. Both reduce one's quality of life by interfering with one's ability to communicate, work, participate in daily activities, and manage stress. Sleep difficulties and sensory sensitivities contribute to fatigue and anger.

Fatigue

Mental/cognitive fatigue and physical fatigue are struggles for survivors of brain injury. Mental fatigue "may result from increased or inefficient cognitive activity when individuals try to sustain or divide attention, deal with simultaneous cognitive tasks, or strive to mentally organize or retrieve information" (Ouellet & Morin, 2006). In the context of TBI, fatigue "may result from the neuronal injury occurring diffusely and in centers mediating arousal, attention, and response speed, including the ascending reticular activating system, limbic system, anterior cingulate, middle frontal, and basal ganglia areas" (Ponsford et al., 2015). Basically, fatigue originates from several areas of the brain, all of which are healing at different rates. Pathological fatigue associated with mild traumatic brain injury

> occurs when the amount of effort required to induce the sense of tiredness or exhaustion, reduced power and motivation is considerably smaller than expected in a healthy individual. Energy resources are depleted more quickly and more extensively than normally expected and pathological fatigue is not as responsive to sleep and rest.
>
> (Norrie et al., 2010)

Ouellet and Morin (2006) found that fatigued survivors of brain injury experienced higher levels of depression, anxiety, cognitive disturbance, and anger/irritability. Participants in their study reported that fatigue interfered with their daily routines, such as eating, personal hygiene, social and leisure activities, mental activity, work, or volunteer tasks, and decreased their quality of life. Their mental fatigue was followed by physical fatigue. One survivor stated that her irritation and agitation increase when she is fatigued. She also stated that fatigue steals her energy. Her coping mechanism is to stop, slow down, and rest. Other studies (Ponsford et al., 2015) have shown that fatigue results from efforts to compensate for cognitive impairments such as slower processing speed and difficulty with attention and vigilance task performance. According to Gronwall et al. (2002), fatigue is the most limiting of the deficits associated with brain injury and may persist for months or years post-injury. The frequency of fatigue among all brain injury severities ranges from 32.4% to 73% (Ponsford, 2013). The injured individual tires more quickly than expected. Activities including simple tasks, concentrating, exercising, or talking contribute to overall fatigue. One survivor (personal communication, January 11, 2012) explained that expending energy is "like bicycling into an invisible wind. Everything seems to take more effort." Another described fatigue as walking through cooked oatmeal. Some survivors stated that, for every family event or social exercise, it takes them two to three days to recover. To watch a movie or television show requires concentration and attention to the characters and story line, all of which is difficult and can cause fatigue.

Studies have shown that generally persons who have suffered a TBI function better during the morning than during the afternoon or evening hours. One survivor stated that noon for her is a normal person's five o'clock in the evening. In the afternoon, she is unable to perform to the level she did in the morning. Some survivors may wake up feeling refreshed, but within a couple of hours, the fatigue sets in making it difficult to carry on with the daily tasks of living. Most of the time, however, an individual with a brain injury does not wake up refreshed because s/he may spend more time in the lighter stages of sleep. So, s/he wakes up with less energy and uses the energy s/he does have more quickly than the normal person. Therefore, if a friend who has a brain injury says that s/he is too tired to go out or complete an activity, s/he is. The common response to fatigue in the general population to is to persevere and to push through to finish the job. But, with brain injury, this approach creates a downward spiral of deterioration, mistakes, and inefficiency. Often, when a person with a brain injury is overtired, s/he can become more talkative, restless, more disorganized and distractable, and less able to reason and can experience increased mood swings. It is important for the family to monitor his/her activities so that they can redirect the survivor before s/he reaches the overtired stage (Gronwall et al., 2002). Signs that the loved one is fatigued "are increasing irritability, unusual pallor, a drawn tense look, or a rather glazed expression in the eyes" (Gronwall et al., 2002).

Fatigue also exaggerates the other deficits from the brain injury. One survivor stated that, when she is fatigued, her balance, judgment, self-awareness, and self-control are impaired. The ability to manage emotions fluctuates with fatigue (Gronwall et al., 2002). Another interesting signal of fatigue is the experience of body temperature changes. Excessive cold "is part of the way that the body signals that it is tired" (Gronwall et al., 2002). I believe that management of fatigue is the key to managing the other deficits of brain injury.

Coping strategies to manage fatigue that I recommend are rest, pace, and quiet. Planning for rest periods during the day helps to manage fatigue. Rest may simply mean closing one's eyes for a few minutes, or it may entail a nap or a time to simply go outside and enjoy nature. Another technique is to learn how to pace one's activities. For example, if the survivor has more energy in the morning, s/he should use that time to tackle more difficult cognitive tasks. After the task is completed, s/he should rest or engage in a less demanding activity. Quiet involves a reduction in external stimulation that can not only distract the survivor but also contribute to premature fatigue. Rest when needed, pace when multiple tasks are required, and quiet to ensure the more successful completion of tasks.

Coping Strategies for Fatigue

Additional compensatory strategies recommended by Sloan and Ponsford (2013) include the following: (1) modify the environment to reduce distractions, (2) train the injured person to identify signs of fatigue and take appropriate action, (3) modify the task to reduce the amount of information to be processed, (4) allow a realistic time frame to complete tasks, and (5) practice stress management, relaxation, or mindfulness exercises. Ouellet and Morin (2006) suggested that effective interventions should be a combination of "gradual physical reconditioning, cognitive restructuring, cognitive training, [a] gradual increase in social or occupational activities, anxiety-reducing strategies, and teaching of proper energy management techniques." Ponsford et al. (2015) recommended modification of the injured person's lifestyle "to restore

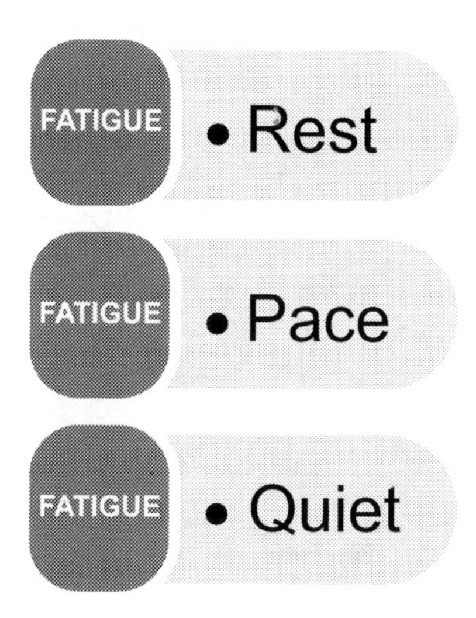

Figure 11.1 Coping strategies for fatigue.

a balance between the demands of the environment and the individual's cognitive and physical capacity."

Sleep

Disturbances in sleep patterns are common in brain injury. Fatigue is one of the most prominent consequences of sleep disorders. Studies have shown that survivors of TBI have a "reduction in sleep efficiency, increased sleep-onset latency, and increased time awake after sleep" (Ponsford et al., 2015). Sleep problems "are associated with negative outcomes (i.e., prolonged impaired cognition, decreased benefit from rehabilitation therapy, and higher cost of care) in acute and postacute stages" (Holcomb et al., 2016b). One brain injury survivor stated that she does not sleep deeply anymore. She said that she is easily awakened and cannot sleep through the night without waking up several times. Insomnia, the difficulty initiating and maintaining sleep, affects 30–70% of individuals with TBI (Ouellet & Morin, 2006). Sleep apnea, a sleep-related breathing disorder characterized by repeated cessation of ventilation during sleep, is estimated to occur in 23–75% of the TBI population (Holcomb et al., 2016a). It is also a risk factor for stroke and a contributing factor to depression (Nakase-Richardson & Schwartz, 2018). A meta-analysis study found that sleep-related breathing disorder "is present in up to 72% of ischemic and hemorrhagic stroke and transient ischemic attack patients" (Holcomb et al., 2016a). Excessive daytime sleepiness is another common complaint, affecting up to 50% of survivors of TBI (Wei et al., 2020). Wei et al. (2020) found that sleep apnea, insomnia, and excessive daytime sleepiness were more prevalent in older adults with TBI in Taiwan than in a similar demographic without TBI.

The practice of good sleep hygiene will help to alleviate the extreme fatigue in survivors of TBI that "may be one of the most important barriers to returning to work or to school, because they can no longer keep up with regular professional or academic schedules that do not allow much time for rest" (Ouellet & Morin, 2006). According to Monden et al. (2018) sleep hygiene consists of four domains: homeostatic factors such as regular exercise; circadian factors such as increased exposure to bright light; medication and drug effects such as restriction of alcohol and caffeine consumption; and arousal in the sleep setting, such as stress management during the day and bedtime rituals. Blue light therapy has been shown to decrease daytime sleepiness and improve cognitive function, sleep quality, and mood.

Anger

Problems with managing anger are common, especially after severe traumatic brain injury. Irritability and aggression are present in "29% to 73% of individuals with traumatic brain injury and are often chronic and pervasive, contributing to social isolation, care burden, disrupted interpersonal relationships, and incomplete community integration" (Hammond et al., 2014). Antonak et al.

(1993) found that anger is worthy of two categories: internalized anger and externalized anger. According to their study, internalized anger is self-directed bitterness and resentment often associated with guilt and self-blame for the injury. Externalized anger is displayed as behavioral disinhibition, irritability, aggressiveness, affective instability, impulsivity, and sexual aggression. Anger outbursts are associated with frustration because of cognitive and physical deficits and are particularly stressful for the family. It is extremely important to educate the family that their loved one is not to blame for the outbursts. It is a result of the brain injury (namely, frontal lobe damage among other areas), not a personal decision or character statement. Early in recovery, the survivor of TBI may say inappropriate or vulgar words with little to no awareness of or control over the behavior. As the individual improves, s/he may have the motivation to participate actively in the therapeutic process of developing coping strategies to control his/her anger. Ponsford (2013) recommended ascertaining a comprehensive history of how the anger manifests, such as yelling, throwing things, or hitting objects or persons. The responses of family members may contribute to the problem, which needs to be addressed. The family should be educated that the anger reaction may be due to the role of a frontolimbic injury to the brain. Also, when the anger is triggered, the injured individual has less ability to reason. Therefore, when families try to communicate with the individual and to understand what is happening, it becomes an agitating factor that escalates the interaction.

Anger may be triggered by increased sensitivity to light, crowds, or loud noises. Additionally, substance use and mood changes negatively contribute to anger control. Ponsford (2013) suggested that the survivor keep a diary of anger outbursts, listing the precipitating factors, thoughts, feelings, reactions from others, and what happened post-outburst. She stated that the record "can be used as a baseline, to identify the circumstances which provoke anger, and ways in which thoughts, feelings, behaviours, and environmental factors including the responses of others can either fuel the anger or have a calming influence." The diary entry provides an educational resource for the person and family on how to avoid triggering outbursts. Some triggers include not being able to follow the conversation, too many conversations at once, pain, feeling too cold or too hot, or fatigue.

Coping strategies for managing anger include deep breathing, walking away, changing the subject, lowering the lights, turning off the television or radio, or going for a walk. McKinlay and Hickox (1988) created an acronym for ANGER management:

A – Anticipate the trigger situations
N – Notice the signs of rising anger
G – Go through the "temper routine" of calming down
E – Extract yourself from the situation
R – Record how you coped, listing lessons that can be employed in the future

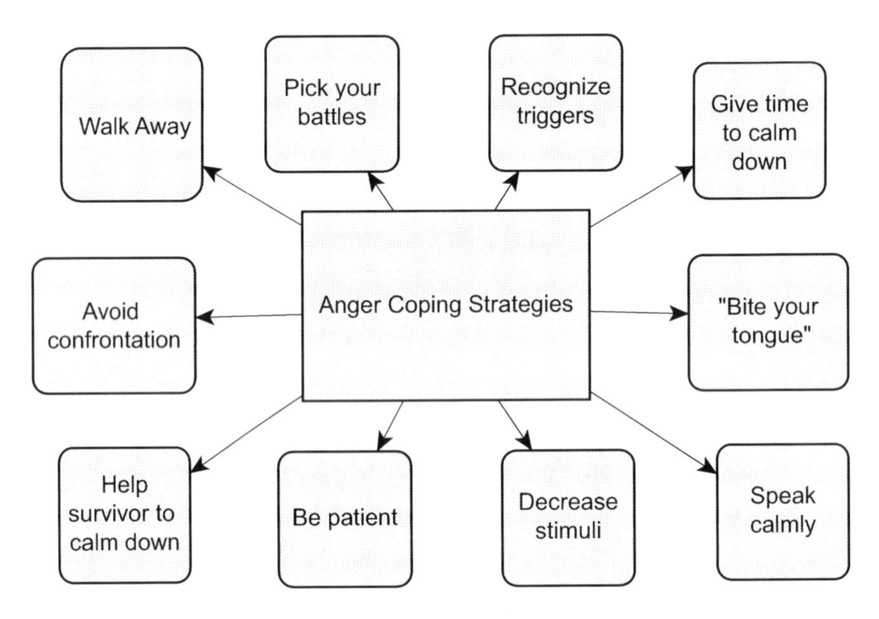

Figure 11.2 Anger coping strategies.

Time-out is another technique that can help to alleviate anger outbursts. This involves the removal of attention by averting one's gaze, walking away for a time, or ignoring the undesirable behavior (Wood, 1984). Daily routines that incorporate choice, access to meaningful activities, and positive communication may avert inappropriate behavior (Ylvisaker et al., 2003). Guidelines suggested by Ponsford (2013) include ignoring angry outbursts by making no direct response. She offered, "[D]o not react to aggression by shouting, arguing, hitting back or becoming upset in front of the injured individual. This will only serve to increase the level of agitation and/or reinforce the behaviour." Respond positively to appropriate behavior and ignore inappropriate behavior. Once the person with a brain injury has calmed down, review what happened and work toward better ways of dealing with the trigger. It is best (although difficult) not to take the outbursts personally, be critical, or hold grudges. The diagram shown in Figure 11.2 highlights some suggestions made by survivors of brain injury that have helped them to manage their anger (Adams, 2012).

Anger Coping Strategies

Adams and Dahdah (2016) found that family members apply different techniques to deal with the anger of their loved one. One caregiver stated that he would let his son "run down like a bad battery." Another loved one stated that she would comment, "I'm sensing this. . . . What's going on?" which helped to reduce the tension. One caregiver voiced to her daughter who had a brain injury that she seemed agitated, but she did not understand why. This opened the door to a conversation in which the daughter felt able to share her agitation in a safe manner. One survivor stated jokingly, "I keep a bag of tongues with me since I bite mine off so often." She also stated that survivors need to be alone when they are agitated or angry. In her opinion, survivors do not need someone to try to fix the problem; rather, they need time to calm down on their own without interference. Voicing that s/he is fatigued helps to alert the family that the loved one has a shorter fuse and to be more aware that s/he is more irritable than usual.

Arciniegas and Wortzel (2019) explained that posttraumatic irritability is more accurately understood as a disorder of affect rather than of mood. They stated that posttraumatic irritability "reflects disturbances of moment-to-moment emotion rather than a persistent change in baseline emotion." Although people with posttraumatic irritability

> are prone to experience and express transient irritation, impatience, anger, and/or loss of temper in response to the events of daily life, their emotional state between episodes of irritation often is relatively neutral (i.e., they do not experience sustained, excessive, and context-independent irritability or anger).

Counseling Considerations

Because of the potential sensory issues, the management of fatigue and anger in the counseling office starts with environmental control. It is recommended that the therapist adjust lighting, noise, and temperature per the needs of the client with a brain injury. For example, I have some clients that cannot handle light at all. So, all lights (overhead and lamps) are turned off. The client is positioned with his/her back against a window to avoid direct light from outside. Another client is unable to handle the white noise machine that drowns out any sounds outside of the office. Some clients can handle a small light but not the sound of a fan. Customization of one's office to alleviate these needs is essential for clients to participate as fully as possible.

Other accommodations include providing shorter sessions to manage fatigue. If possible, schedule counseling sessions in the morning hours, outside of rush hour traffic. Adjusting the room's temperature may also help to alleviate or stave off fatigue and anger. One client may experience a "hot flash" when fatigued, while another may become very cold. The therapist needs to be aware of the specific signs of fatigue exhibited by each client and modify the environment as necessary.

Another technique that I employ is commending the client for his/her effort and attention to the counseling process. Acknowledging his/her energy output and appreciating his/her desire to participate to the best of his/her ability goes a long way toward helping him/her know that the counselor recognizes the cost for them to come to a session. This also models to their family how to encourage and appreciate the small things that a person with brain injury recognizes cost them greatly in energy and resources. Last, if possible, establish a routine standing appointment so that the person with brain injury can depend on that day and time for each session. This reduces the possibility that s/he will forget the appointment and the irritation of having to remember a different counseling time from appointment to appointment.

Cognitive-Behavioral Therapy

Cognitive-behavioral therapy (CBT) has been established as a useful model for managing fatigue and anger in the general population. Because of its success, it is recommended as a therapy technique for the brain injury population. Neumann et al. (2017) found that survivors of TBI were more likely to interpret others' behavior as intentional, hostile, and blameworthy than participants without a TBI. The more intentionally hostile and blameworthy a participant believed a situation to be, the angrier they became. Neumann et al. recommended CBT "to reframe the maladaptive thoughts that a person has about oneself, others, or their surrounding environment to reduce subsequent unpleasant emotional responses." They stated that unwarranted negative attributions are cognitive distortions that should be restructured.

According to Demark and Gemeinhardt (2002), "a complete understanding of the person's cognitive status is necessary before embarking on any kind of intervention for anger, as well as a thorough knowledge of their overall social and adaptive functioning." Cognitive therapy and cognitive-behavioral therapy are recommended to help survivors of brain injury manage their anger. The goal is to increase the client's awareness of thought patterns and cognitive distortions and to teach a way to manage emotional responses. As mentioned earlier, it is a good idea for the survivor to keep a diary of anger episodes and thought records as a means of managing automatic beliefs that affect mood. The identification of problem-solving techniques may be helpful to assist the injured individual create new strategies to address problems. Demark and Gemeinhardt (2002) recommended role play as a means of problem-solving in a safe environment.

Dahdah et al. (2018) stated that cognitive-behavioral therapy for insomnia (CBTi) is a suggested standard by the American Academy of Sleep Medicine (AASM). The components of CBTi are sleep education, sleep hygiene, stimulus control, sleep restriction, relaxation, and cognitive therapy. Education on normal sleep processes and information about co-morbid conditions assists with understanding the facets of insomnia. Sleep hygiene consists of creating behaviors that promote sleep and eliminating behaviors that interfere with sleep, for example, creating a routine of relaxation before going to bed, such as taking a hot bath, drinking tea, or reading a book. Elimination of behaviors such as screen (technology) activities, physical exercise, or highly emotional conversations or television programs contributes to winding down before bed. Stimulus control is limiting activities that are not designated for sleep in the bed/bedroom. Sleep restriction reduces the amount of time spent in bed when not asleep. Relaxation includes diaphragmatic breathing, biofeedback, progressive muscle relaxation, visual imagery, and meditation. Cognitive therapy addresses factors contributing to insomnia such as anxiety or worry. It also helps people replace maladaptive sleep-related beliefs (Dahdah et al., 2018).

Christian Counseling

The Bible addresses ways in which to manage fatigue and anger. One of the verses I refer to is James 1:19 (NLT), which says, "Understand this, my dear brothers and sisters: You must all be quick to listen, slow to speak, and slow to get angry." Being quick to listen and slow to speak are two techniques that can help when one is triggered. They also give the listener time to process what is being said and determine whether s/he is understanding the meaning correctly. One survivor of TBI stated that this verse helped him to not act out his anger and irritability as often. Another client shared that she has this verse posted on her mirror at home to help her reduce impulsivity. Proverbs 19:11 (ESV) says, "Good sense makes one slow to anger, and it is his glory to overlook an offense." This verse recommends the reader to overlook an offense or a negative comment. Doing so is very difficult for survivors of brain injury due to the impulsivity that comes with irritability. However, if the therapist can provide another way of looking at the issue and remind him/her that it is possible to overlook an offense, it gives the survivor another way to manage irritability. Proverbs 15:18 (ESV) offers the same coping strategy. It says, "A hot-tempered man stirs up strife, but he who is slow to anger quiets contention." This is also true for the family member who gets triggered by his/her injured loved one. It is best to not engage in an argument because it tends to make matters worse. The alternative to anger and irritability lies in Ephesians 4:31–32 (ESV), which says, "Let all bitterness and wrath and anger and clamor and slander be put away from you, along with all malice. Be kind to one another, tenderhearted, forgiving one another, as God in Christ forgave you." The alternative to anger is love, mercy, and graciousness. 1 Corinthians 13:4–5 (ESV) says, "Love is patient and kind; love does not envy or boast; is not arrogant or rude. It does not insist on its own way; it is not irritable or resentful." And Psalm 103:8 (ESV) says, "The Lord is merciful and gracious, slow to anger and abounding in steadfast love." These last two verses are foundational to overcoming the outbursts that anger and irritability can create. Understanding that there is a different, more productive way of expressing one's emotions can direct the steps of the injured person toward more healthy relationships.

The level of recovery for the person with brain injury determines his/her ability to engage in more positive experiences. For example, early in recovery, the survivor is not aware and not able to recognize how s/he is coming across or the impact of what s/he is saying. As the brain begins to heal, s/he becomes more aware of others. Further in the healing process, it is possible for the person with brain injury to be sensitive to his/her loved ones. Most clients are referred to outpatient counseling from a rehabilitation facility or after they have been home for a few months or years. Typically, these are clients making long-term adjustments to their brain injury. By this time, many caretakers have been fully extended, are burned out, or are on their way to exhaustion. The result is frustration, anger, and irritability not only from the survivor but also from the family member or caretaker. A technique that I use is to normalize their feelings while encouraging them to practice graciousness in their pursuit of self-care and other care. One way of normalizing their feelings is to say, "Brain injury has become another member of the family. At this time, he is making himself fully known. As your loved one improves, brain injury will alternate as a background player instead of the main actor." Most people easily agitated are simply depleted. The same can be said for fatigue. Practicing basic self-care can reduce the spikes in temper and fatigue. Figures 11.3 and 11.4 show the various self-care practices that survivors and families have suggested (Adams, 2012).

If they follow the Christian faith, they are open to God's model in relationships from the scriptures noted earlier. Prayer helps to reinforce these practices and helps to guide the survivor and family members to respond with mercy and love when agitation appears. Helping the survivor to acknowledge the help and love of his/her caretaker goes a long way in helping mend fractures caused by anger and irritation. Most caretakers want to be appreciated for their sacrifices, realizing that the survivor may never really know the full extent of those efforts. However, making strides toward merciful and loving behavior contributes to the survivor performing well in interpersonal relationships and improving his/her family experiences.

Although God Himself modeled the role of resting, it is very difficult for most caregivers to give themselves permission to rest after days and weeks of taking care of their loved one with a brain injury. Exodus 31:17 (ESV) says,

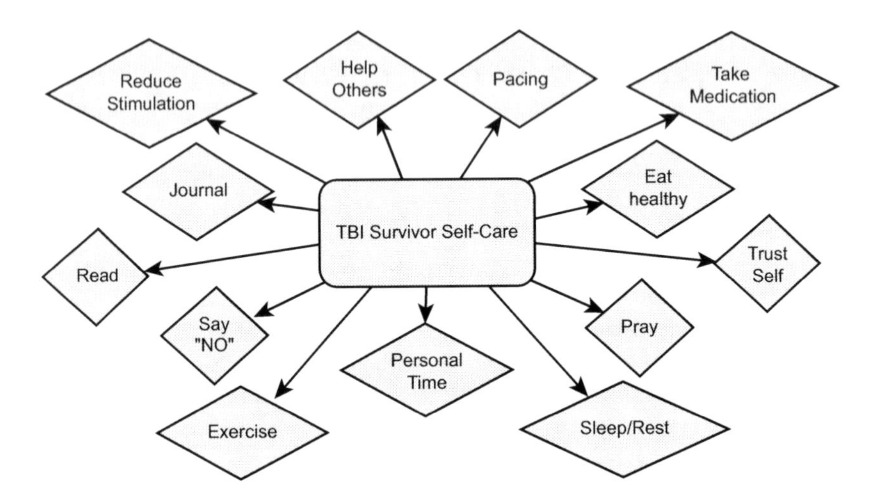

Figure 11.3 Self-care for survivors.

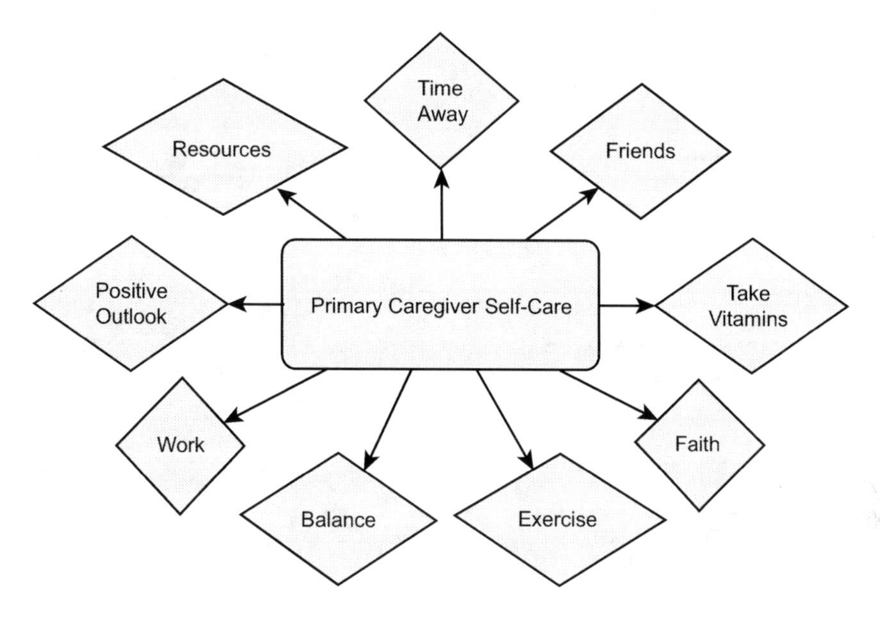

Figure 11.4 Self-care for primary caregivers.

"It is a sign forever between me and the people of Israel that in six days the Lord made heaven and earth, and on the seventh he rested and was refreshed." Often, caregivers focus solely on the survivor, forgetting that rest leads to feeling refreshed and the ability to go again the next day. In my practice, caregivers and family members who were type A personalities before the injury tend to expect recovery to occur in the same manner and speed. Unfortunately, brain injury does not recover at that pace. However, waiting and watching are two of the most effective ways to manage fatigue. Isaiah 40:31 (ESV) says, "But they who wait for the Lord shall renew their strength; they shall mount up with wings like eagles; they shall run and not be weary; they shall walk and not faint." The gift of neuroplasticity is that the brain heals in its own time. Brain injury recovery is not seen minute-by-minute but often month-by-month. Therefore, it is ok to stop, slow down, pace, and rest. Isaiah 58:11 (ESV) holds another promise for Christians. It says, "And the Lord will guide you continually and satisfy your desire in scorched places and make your bones strong; and you will be like a watered garden, like a spring of water, whose waters do not fail." Dependence on God's strength and His provision will relieve the inner pressure to do it all on one's own. Fatigue for the survivor serves a greater purpose when it leads to sleep. It allows the brain to utilize the glymphatic system, which works only in sleep to clear toxins from the brain. In wakefulness, it is disengaged. If one can recognize the benefit of rest, pace, mercy, love, and graciousness, practicing these strategies will improve relationships and the recovery process of brain injury.

Faith and Non-Faith Counseling

Management of anger in the Muslim faith encourages the believer to seek refuge in Allah. Retreat to silence, not moving, and changing positions (i.e., from sitting to lying down) are three suggestions in dealing with anger. According to the Prophet Mohammad, the control of anger gives one a higher status and exalted character. Also, asking for gratitude assuages anger. The Jewish faith suggests that the path to move away from anger is to cultivate humility. Humble people do not feel the need to insult others to feel good about themselves. They can shrug off insults as having no basis in reality. Humility releases one from the worry of what others think. Additionally, the Jewish faith states that anger can be dispelled by emphasizing the love of God and joy in following the commandments. Attendance at a spiritual service as a means of being alone with Allah or God can help to reduce agitation and heighten a calm spirit.

If the client does not subscribe to a certain faith, assisting him/her to recognize the role of anger in his/her life is helpful. In other words, help him/her to see the irritation and agitation as clues to help him/her recognize what is out of balance in his/her world. Is there a reason it is coming up now? What is the anger trying to say? If it were a map, where would it direct one? It is helpful to see fatigue in the same light. What is fatigue trying to say? What is out of balance? Instead of avoiding the feelings, encourage the survivor to use them as signs that can highlight what is wrong and direct healthy behavior. Deep breathing helps to decrease the fast heart rate of anger and invites a sense of calm that can reduce fatigue. Last, assign a trusted friend or family member to help the survivor recognize judgment errors. For example, if a survivor takes a comment negatively, the friend can help him/her know what the comment really meant. If the survivor is fatigued, the trusted friend can direct him/her to rest or slow down. An accountability partner creates space for other caregivers to live their lives and creates a springboard for the survivor to begin to trust his/her own brain after the injury.

Conclusion

Two of the most difficult deficits of brain injury are anger and fatigue. They both contribute to lower quality of life and poor use of energy resources. This chapter discussed the contributors of anger and fatigue from both the survivor and caregiver perspective. Sleep hygiene and various therapeutic exercises including self-care were presented. Management of anger and fatigue from Christian, faith, and non-faith perspectives addressed various strategies to cope with these deficits. The final chapter addresses the role of self-concept and purpose. Strategies to regain one's personhood and develop a purpose after brain injury are highlighted.

References

Adams, D. (2012). *Coping strategies of traumatic brain injury survivors and primary caregivers.* [Unpublished doctoral dissertation]. B.H. Carroll Theological Institute.

Adams, D. & Dahdah, M. (2016). Coping and adaptive strategies of traumatic brain injury survivors and primary caregivers. *Journal of NeuroRehabilitation, 39*(2), 223–237.

Antonak, R., Livneh, H., & Antonak, C. (1993). A review of research on psychosocial adjustment to impairment in persons with traumatic brain injury. *Journal of Head Trauma Rehabilitation, 8*(4), 87–100.

Arciniegas, D., & Wortzel, H. (2019). Emotional dyscontrol. In J. Silver, T. McAllister, & D. Arciniegas (Eds.), *Textbook of Traumatic Brain Injury* (3rd ed., pp. 347–360). American Psychiatric Association Publishing.

Dahdah, M., Bell, K., Lequerica, A., & Merfeld, A. (2018). Effectiveness of cognitive behavioral therapy for treating insomnia in healthy individuals and those with brain injury. *Brain Injury Professional, 14*(4), 12–14.

Demark, J., & Gemeinhardt, M. (2002). Anger and it's management for survivors of acquired brain injury. *Brain Injury, 16*(2), 91–108. https://doi.org/10.1080/02699050110102059

Gronwall, D., Wrightson, P., & Waddell, P. (2002). *Head injury: The facts* (2nd ed.). Oxford University Press.

Hammond, F., Bickett, A., Norton, J., & Pershad, R. (2014). Effectiveness of amantadine hydrochloride in the reduction of chronic traumatic brain injury irritability and aggression. *Journal of Head Trauma Rehabilitation, 29*(5), 391–399.

Holcomb, E., Schwartz, D., McCarthy, M., Thomas, B., Barnett, S., & Nakase-Richardson, R. (2016a). Incidence, characterization, and predictors of sleep apnea in consecutive brain injury rehabilitation admissions. *Journal of Head Trauma Rehabilitation, 31*(2), 82–100.

Holcomb, E., Towns, S., Kamper, J., Barnett, S., Sherer, M., Evans, C., & Nakase-Richardson, R. (2016b). The relationship between sleep-wake cycle disturbance and trajectory of cognitive recovery during acute traumatic brain injury. *Journal of Head Trauma Rehabilitation, 31*(2), 108–116.

McKinlay, W., & Hickox, A. (1988). How can families help in the rehabilitation of the head injured? *Journal of Head Trauma Rehabilitation, 3*(4), 64–72.

Monden, K., Gerber, D., Newman, J., Philippus, A., Biggs, J., Schneider, H., Spier, E., Weintraub, A., & Makley, M. (2018). Sleep hygiene: A novel, nonpharmacological approach to treating sleep-wake cycle disturbance after moderate to severe brain injury on an inpatient rehabilitation unit. *Brain Injury Professional, 14*(4), 20–21.

Nakase-Richardson, R., & Schwartz, D. (2018). Sleep apnea and traumatic brain injury. *Brain Injury Professional, 14*(4), 8–10.

Neumann, D., Malec, J., & Hammond, F. (2017). Negative attribution bias and anger after traumatic brain injury. *Journal of Head Trauma Rehabilitation, 32*(3), 197–204.

Norrie, J., Heitger, M., Leathem, J., Anderson, T., Jones, R., & Flett, R. (2010). Mild traumatic brain injury and fatigue: A prospective longitudinal study. *Brain Injury, 24*(13–14), 1528–1538. https://doi.org/10.3109/02699052.2010.531687

Ouellet, M., & Morin, C. (2006). Fatigue following traumatic brain injury: Frequency, characteristics, and associated factors. *Rehabilitation Psychology, 51*(2), 140–149. https://doi.org/10.1037/0090-5550.51.2.140

Ponsford, J. (2013). Mechanism, recovery and sequelae of traumatic brain injury: A foundation for the REAL approach. In J. Ponsford, S. Sloan, & P. Snow (Eds.), *Traumatic brain injury: Rehabilitation for everyday adaptive living* (2nd ed., pp. 1–33). Psychology Press.

Ponsford, J. (2013). Dealing with the impact of TBI on psychological adjustment and relationships. In J. Ponsford, S. Sloan, & P. Snow (Eds.), *Traumatic brain injury: Rehabilitation for everyday adaptive living* (2nd ed., pp. 226–262). Psychology Press.

Ponsford, J. (2013). Assessment and management of behaviour problems. In J. Ponsford, S. Sloan, & P. Snow (Eds.), *Traumatic brain injury: Rehabilitation for everyday adaptive living* (2nd ed., pp. 164–191). Psychology Press.

Ponsford, J., Schönberger, M., & Rajaratnam, S. (2015). A model of fatigue following traumatic brain injury. *Journal of Head Trauma Rehabilitation, 30*(4), 277–282.

Sloan, S., & Ponsford, J. (2013). Managing cognitive problems following TBI. In J. Ponsford, S. Sloan, & P. Snow (Eds.), *Traumatic brain injury: Rehabilitation for everyday adaptive living* (2nd ed., pp. 99–132). Psychology Press.

Wei, L., Wen, Y., Thompson, H., Liu, C., Su, Y., Chen, P., Chen, C., Chuang, Y., Lin, Y., Chen, C., Chen, C., Chiu, H., & Chiu, H. (2020). Sleep disturbances following traumatic brain injury in older adults: A comparison study. *Journal of Head Trauma Rehabilitation, 35*(4), 288–295.

Wood, R. (1984). Behaviour disorders following severe brain injury: Their presentation and psychological management. In N. Brooks (Ed.), *Closed head injury: Psychological, social and family consequences* (pp. 195–219). Oxford University Press.

Ylvisaker, M., Jacobs, H., & Feeney, T. (2003). Positive supports for people who experience behavioral and cognitive disability after brain injury: A review. *Journal of Head Trauma Rehabilitation, 18*(1), 7–32.

12 Counseling Self-Concept and Purpose

Case Study

Robbie was a young, 30-year-old executive with a software company. He had recently graduated with a master's degree in business and was living independently in Washington, where he moved for his job. One evening, Robbie and his brother, who was visiting from out of state, were to meet for dinner at a local pub. While looking at his cell phone, Robbie walked onto the crosswalk as directed by the light and was hit from behind by a taxi. His body hit the windshield and rolled onto the pavement. Robbie suffered a severe traumatic brain injury along with multiple fractures and contusions. An ambulance was summoned to the scene, which found him unresponsive and unconscious. He was transported to a local trauma hospital where his body was in a coma for five weeks. Because Robbie's parents lived in a different state, they requested that he be transferred to their local rehabilitation facility when he was well enough to be transported. Waking from the coma, Robbie did not remember the accident. He was unable to recall where he worked or what he did. Nothing made sense to him. An accountant by trade, Robbie was unable to compute simple math problems. He had to relearn how to walk, eat, drink, and perform activities of daily living. His parents and brothers were at his side during the long recovery. Eventually, Robbie was able to participate in residential rehabilitation where he stayed for several months. Once discharged, he moved in with his parents where he lives today. It has been over ten years since the accident, and Robbie has found meaningful activities with volunteer work. Although he states that he would like to return to work, he understands that he is not yet capable of managing the responsibilities of a part-time or full-time job. Instead, Robbie volunteers with a local disability organization, participates in church activities, studies math, exercises, reads, journals, and helps care for his parents, who both have compromised health. Robbie's brothers live close to them, which is very helpful when he feels overwhelmed. Although he struggles with his temper at times, he remembers to "not lose his manners" and tries to go to his room to quiet down. His brother stated that he feels guilty because he should have been there to keep his brother from being hit by the taxi. Robbie reminds him to not feel guilty. He states that he is happy and feels as though God has given him

DOI: 10.4324/9781003301912-12

an opportunity to help so many people who are disadvantaged or disabled. He enjoys his volunteer work and believes that he is contributing to society in a unique way. Robbie also has a strong faith and believes that God has him here for a purpose . . . and it is not to be a software accountant.

Overview

William Winslade (1998) stated that being human is not just the organic function of one's body. He said, "Being persons requires having a personality, being aware of ourselves and our surroundings, and possessing human capacities, such as memory, emotions, and the ability to communicate and interact with other people." When someone has a brain injury, these ingredients of humanity may be damaged or limited, but it does not forfeit one's claim to personhood. He continued, "When we give brain-injury victims the care they need to save their lives but withhold the care they need to reach their potential, we compound the initial tragedy." As a society, Winslade recommended restoring the virtues of empathy, compassion, fairness, and civility. Nurturing and maintaining those virtues in the hospital and in the home create the environment for optimum recovery for the survivor of brain injury and his/her family. Lennon et al. (2014) stated that an acquired brain injury catapults the individual to reconstruct his/her sense of self, and that the reconstruction is complicated by the ongoing cognitive, emotional, and behavioral difficulties associated with the injury. The loss of self refers to a sense of grief and longing for the pre-injury self, and reconstructing the self refers to the process of rebuilding a new post-injury identity. An expanding sense of self after brain injury has been described as

> feeling as though one was given a second chance at life, focusing on short-term goals and a desire for stable outcomes in terms of employment and relationships, taking a positive meaning from their experience, re-evaluating priorities and weighting social norms of success as less important and inner successes as more important.
>
> (Lennon et al., 2014)

Lennon et al. (2014) found that individuals with acquired brain injury believed that engaging in meaningful activity (engaging with the external world in some capacity) has a positive influence in reconstructing their sense of self. Meaningful, productive activity "is key to developing life satisfaction and a sense of contribution to society, and often provides an avenue for social interaction" (Payne et al., 2018). In some studies, occupational value generates a sense of meaning (Nyman et al., 2021). The sense of meaning is connected to one's purpose in life as it pertains to relationships, rediscovering oneself, and envisioning future possibilities (Olofsson et al., 2020). However difficult and monumental a brain injury is, it is not prohibitive of developing a healthy self-concept and meaningful life.

Self-Concept

The term self-concept may be described in different ways and may also entail similar ideas, such as self-efficacy and self-esteem. Douglas (2013) defined self-concept as a "multi-dimensional, internal representation of the individual." It consists of thoughts and feelings and of how one perceives oneself in relation to one's values and experiences.Vickery et al. (2006) explained that self-concept is a

> collection of beliefs about an individual's own functioning in various life dimensions, such as physical self-concept and social self-concept, and is seen as an apparatus that permits self-reflection, allows individuals to regulate their behavior by providing motivation to select and work toward goals, and underlies all perceptions, beliefs, and feelings about oneself.

After TBI, self-concept is altered.The changes occur dynamically "as the person develops awareness of the consequences of the injury and adapts to new experiences and challenges" (Knox et al., 2017).

The role of decision-making may contribute to the development of self-concept post-injury. Knox et al. (2017) explored the connection between self-concept and decision-making in the lives of survivors of severe traumatic brain injury.They found that there is a relationship between an individual's goals and his/her self-concept after injury. Goals may be seen as "both arising [from] and contributing to self-concept." Knox et al. also studied the relationship between decision-making, goal-setting, and self-conceptualization. The participants in their study believed that goals motivated them to make decisions, thus making them more autonomous. Making decisions helped them to feel more in control of their lives, which contributed to their self-concept post-injury.

The role of friends and families is key to self-concept. Knox et al. (2017) stated that friends and family could provide a "buffer against negative social comparisons and provide feedback that supported participants to recognize their achievements" (Knox et al., 2017). Understanding brain injury and its implications helps families feel more confident and competent in serving their loved ones (Waldron-Perrine et al., 2019). In Knox et al.'s (2017) study, four suggestions were made describing appropriate types of support: (1) create decision-making opportunities, (2) provide expert advice, (3) act on behalf of the loved one with a brain injury, and (4) motivate and provide encouragement. Robbie's dad (in the case study presented earlier) stated that his main contribution was to encourage and support his son at every step of his progress.

The sense of self is key to the recovery and adaptation process after a brain injury. Fadyl et al. (2019) recommended that if the sense of self "is acknowledged appropriately and the process of dealing with changes is supported positively, this could powerfully enable people in developing and maintaining resources that help them recover from and live with TBI." Self-esteem has been defined as "a self-evaluative process in which an individual judges him- or herself either negatively or positively, based on personal abilities and attributes" (Klonoff, 2010). Like self-concept, self-esteem has been considered a mediator of improved psychosocial functioning and adjustment to brain injury. In general, self-efficacy has been defined as "personal belief in one's capability to organize and execute actions in striving for various attainment" (Klonoff, 2010). She also stated that the combination of self-esteem and mastery creates "inner contentment, enthusiasm, positive affect, creativity, goodwill, and the appreciation of one's circumstances."

Return to Work

Community integration involves four constructs: occupational activity, social relationships, independent living skills, and assimilation into the community (Winkler et al., 2006). Obtaining and maintaining employment is associated with well-being and quality of life and therefore is one of the most important goals post-injury (Tsaousides et al., 2009). Failure to return to one's pre-injury work or academic ability "is one of the most devastating consequences of traumatic brain injury, contributing directly to a decrease in psychosocial adjustment and to a deterioration in the quality of life of the entire family group, not just the survivor" (Cattelani et al., 2002). Studies have shown that unemployment rates after TBI range from 18% to 88% (Tsaousides et al., 2009). Shigaki et al. (2009) found that "only 38% of participants with TBI were in the work force at 2-years post-injury, with a concurrent 22% increase in unemployment over baseline." They also found that the "average reported income from earned sources declined 51%, while mean monthly public assistance increased 275%." So, there are "estimated national losses of $642 million for lost wages, $96 million in lost income and $353 million in increased public assistance in the first year post-TBI." Hoofien et al. (2001) found that 58.6% of the participants in their study reported that their main source of income was compensatory allowance and 13.7% reported a salary, while 4% relied on family support and 23.7% reported various combinations of these. The types of employment in this study were lower-level technology and administration jobs that involved a structured routine, with little room for creativity or initiation and limited interpersonal interaction. Employment is defined as "engagement in gainful work activities" and is associated with quality of life (Tsaousides et al., 2009). However, when the survivor returns to work, it is unclear whether the individual was able to return to the same job, the same hours worked, and/or the same level of responsibility. In Australia, Hawthorne et al. (2009) found that 35% of the participants with TBI were working at a job at a lower level, 51% at the same level, and 14% at a higher level. Interestingly, their study outcome did not appear to be related to the severity of the brain injury. Studies have shown that feelings of success and failure are strongly influenced by the subjective experience of the survivor as it pertains to his/her "personal values, beliefs regarding employment, and self-appraisals of productivity, rather than traditional measures of job productivity, such as hours worked or salary earned" (Tsaousides et al., 2009). In other words, part-time or volunteer work may be considered worthwhile regardless of the salary or lack of salary. Bandura (1977) defined self-efficacy as the belief in one's ability to perform a particular task to successfully attain a future goal. So, employment-related self-efficacy is the individual's "belief in his or her ability to find a job or to carry out work-related tasks successfully" (Tsaousides et al., 2009). These researchers found that self-efficacy was a better predictor of quality of life than employment status.

Recommendations for Return to Work

When the survivor of brain injury is ready to return to work, there are accommodations that may be put in place to maximize success. Kreutzer and Sander (1997) outlined compensatory strategies for a survivor of TBI. They suggested that the employee (1) negotiate with his/her employer a reasonable number of new responsibilities, and a slow, progressive addition of responsibilities; (2) organize his/her desk and workspace for optimum efficiency; (3) learn to react calmly and assertively to unreasonable assignments; and (4) reach out to a job coach or vocational rehabilitation therapist for stress management techniques. Work adaptations to manage sensory issues have also been recommended (Donker-Cools et al., 2018). For example, the employer may allow the survivor to work from home or to have a separate office in which s/he can control the light, temperature, and external noise. To reduce eye fatigue, the employee may be provided an anti-glare matte screen for the computer monitor. One survivor stated that she did not want a phone on her desk but preferred to be emailed any directives or information. This avoided the noise of a ringing telephone and gave her time to process the written communication. Notepads should be available for the survivor to writing notes to compensate for short-term memory issues. Another survivor asked for (and was granted) a place to nap when he experienced cognitive fatigue. This kept the employee at the office and gave him time to rest and refresh before tackling another work assignment. A separate work area may also reduce interruptions from colleagues and prevent organic conversations, which tend to be exhausting for survivors of brain injury. Last, adjusted work hours to avoid rush hour traffic will prevent the survivor from being fatigued before s/he begins his/her workday. One client's employer gave him leeway to work part-time at first and slowly moved him to full-time status.

Resilience

A common characteristic that describes survivors of brain injury is their resilience. The strength that comes from facing and advancing despite adversity has been an admirable trait for many survivors. Resilience has been described as "personal qualities and skills that enable a person to adapt well in the face of adversity or trauma" (Waldron-Perrine et al., 2019). It is known to be associated with lower distress, fewer symptoms, improved functional outcomes, and better quality of life for individuals recovering from brain injury. Iverson (2012) stated that resilience "is an intrinsic characteristic underlying a person's ability to successfully adapt to acute stress and more chronic forms of adversity." He also said that the possible underpinnings of resilience are facing fears, adaptive coping, optimism and positive emotions, positive reframing and acceptance, social competence, and purpose in life. Godwin and Kreutzer (2013) identified factors that highlight the role of resilience in the rehabilitation process. They recommended that resilience be addressed at both the individual and family levels to normalize emotional responses and maximize emotional communication to facilitate families working together; to help individuals focus on post-injury gains instead of pre-injury functioning; and to develop new goals to achieve success. Facilitation and maintenance of hope with an emphasis on abilities and strengths versus limitations and disabilities undergird the resilience needed for optimum recovery. Waldron-Perrine et al. (2019) recommended that therapists place an "emphasis on maintaining hope in the context of preparing individuals and families for acceptance of some significant life and functional changes." They stated that "individuals who overcome and achieve goals beyond typical recovery expectations may be the individuals with the most resilience, personal drive, and ambition." Cicerone (1989) believed that the therapist working with a client with brain injury should deal with the issues associated the injury while providing realistic estimates of the client's future, "without precluding the possibility of change and taking away the patient's hope and motivation."

Benefit-finding is a coping mechanism used to encourage resiliency. Helping the survivor to recognize the idea of receiving strength and benefit from their adversity has been found to facilitate adaptation and adjustment for recovery (Emmons & McCullogh, 2003). When asked how she coped with the atrocities of Auschwitz, Holocaust and brain injury survivor Rosa Blum explained, "I wanted to see who won. We won. Israel became a nation. I have a family with two sons and three grandchildren and Hitler is dead" (personal conversation February 14, 2018). Resilience "includes the ability to recognize and overcome challenges, manage one's injury and health, and find optimal solutions to problems through a positive lifestyle and outlook" (Waldron-Perrine et al., 2019). Klonoff (2010) believed that resiliency and adaptive coping improve self-esteem, social reintegration, work resumption, and quality of life.

Purpose

To re-create one's life after brain injury requires a renewed purpose. Many survivors of brain injury ask themselves why they lived despite the injury. One survivor stated that her purpose was to offer inspiration and to encourage others to not give up. Others want to educate the public about the effects of brain injury and what they have learned. Another aspect of purpose is to be intentional about laying hold of every moment. Patti Foster states that, since her wreck, she lives with the urgency to not let an opportunity pass. She shares Galatians 6:9–10 (NIV):

> Let us not become weary in doing good, for at the proper time we will reap a harvest if we do not give up. Therefore, as we have opportunity, let us do good to all people, especially to those who belong to the family of believers.

Her mother states that God was not through with her and that it was only through God that she was able to get through her daughter's injury because she wanted to turn and run. Today, she speaks at events with her daughter, sharing God's hope and comfort that they experienced throughout the recovery process. An English teacher who was forced to retire after three brain injuries eventually found her purpose in tutoring students. She stated that God knew her heart was in teaching and that He would lead her back to the classroom. Another survivor stated that she keeps her eyes on what she can do, not on what she cannot do. She believes that this gives her space to search for her passion and pursue those opportunities. Many survivors have volunteered with their local brain injury associations, providing a resource to others who have also struggled with the same issues.

Counseling Considerations

Therapists may contribute to their clients' purpose by helping them to formulate and move toward life goals that align with their self-concept and values. Positive relationships provide "a vehicle for participants to re-establish autonomy and exercise control in their lives" (Knox et al., 2017). These friends and families need to be informed about brain injury and be willing to advocate for their loved one as s/he makes decisions, rather than taking on the role of substitute decision-makers. It is important to invite family and caregivers into the counseling process in order to educate them and to model proper communication and support for their injured loved ones.

Understanding the client's personal sense of spirituality and belief system helps the therapist direct his/her conversations toward establishing personally meaningful goals with the client. Krych and Schmidt (2015) stated that it is critical that those working with clients post-injury prepare them for "a lifelong process of re-creating their lives, finding joy and meaningfulness, and seeking what they need." Helping clients to develop an outlook that there are possibilities for life after brain injury encourages them beyond the limitations of the injury. Additionally, "the therapist's attitude of caring and empathic understanding toward making the person whole are probably of greatest therapeutic value to the survivor of a traumatic brain injury" (Cicerone, 1989).

Psychotherapy

According to Cicerone (1989), a goal of psychotherapy is to increase the client's capacity for self-observation. This may compensate for the loss of internalized self-monitoring. He continued, "particular attention can be paid to exploring and defining the patient's efficacy expectations (i.e., the patient's beliefs regarding their ability to execute specific behaviors leading to desired outcomes)." Cicerone (1989) espoused Prigatano and colleagues' psychotherapeutic model for brain injury, which includes psychoeducation about brain injury; helping the client to deal with the meaning of the injury, to achieve a sense of self-acceptance and forgiveness, to make realistic goals regarding work and relationships, and to behave appropriately in social situations; providing specific behavioral strategies to compensate for deficits; and fostering a realistic sense of hope. The ultimate goal is for the clients to reestablish a sense of meaning in their lives. The therapist must demonstrate that his/her client with brain injury is "accepted for who they are as well as for who they may become" (Cicerone, 1989). Acceptance of who the person is post-injury helps survivors to reach some level of peace, which may decrease anger and increase productivity in daily life. The therapist needs to recognize the emotional impact of the relationship the client has with the therapist in the absence of overt acknowledgment. Tasks and therapeutic assignments are intended to promote greater autonomy and accountability for the client. Goal-setting, self-reliance, and recognition of improvements enhance self-concept (Klonoff, 2010). Elbaum (2007) stated that a sense of control and empowerment increased a client's self-concept and contributed to him actively engaging in his care. This can be attained by "a goal-oriented approach, weaving significant others actively into the process, reinforcing strategies to improve mood and frustration tolerance, as well as ensuring that the survivor is on a productive path emotionally and socially" (Elbaum, 2007). The productive path may include community reintegration, volunteer work, a return to school, or any meaningful activity.

Non-Faith-Based Counseling

For those who do not practice religion, nature has been a source of meaning and purpose. Enjoying the trees and flowers, watching plants grow and bloom, and listening to the birds remind some of the sanctity and meaning of life. Viktor Frankl (1968), a survivor of the Holocaust who created logotherapy, stated that, when all is stripped away, one still can choose one's attitude. He recommends that clients minimize the emphasis on being a victim and rather find meaning for their future life.

When religion is not an active part of someone's life, it is helpful to appeal to his/her sense of ethics. Once an individual identifies his/her core values, the foundation is laid to build a new life and find purpose. Ruff and Chester (2014) suggested that regardless of whether someone is religious, s/he should take direction, support, and comfort from his/her own belief system. Core values may incorporate truth, kindness, contribution, humility, justice, and love. These values create a plumb line from which one can build meaningful activity and purposeful living. If a person keeps a balanced perspective, it will allow him/her to acknowledge deficits while taking responsibility for creating meaning despite, the injury. Ruff and Chester (2014) shared that survivors of brain injury can speak the truth, love, be fair, have courage, and contribute despite their hardships. They can experience gratitude for those individuals, in the past or the present, who have assisted them in some way in their recovery.

Christian and Faith-Based Counseling

Chen (1997) suggested that spirituality and religious faith can help an individual to cope with adversity and limitations through creating a meaningful life and relationship with the world. Spirituality can become "a powerful source of sustenance by providing a rubric for the transformative experience, and thus enabling a patient to make sense of apparently nonsensical losses" (Klonoff, 2010). Johnstone et al. (2009) stated that survivors utilized religious and spiritual resources to cope with their disability and to give new meaning to their lives. Johnstone et al. (2009) divided religious concepts into three categories: spiritual experiences, such as feelings of connectedness with a higher power; religious practices, such as prayer, meditation, and reading; and congregational support, such as social support from fellow congregants. Their research showed that spiritual experiences and congregational support, but not necessarily religious practices, contributed to improved physical and mental health of survivors. Some studies have found that reading scripture gives survivors peace and comfort, as well as does their relationship with God. A survivor of TBI stated that she is trying to make peace with who she is post-injury. Another survivor stated that she was always a believer but, since her brain injury, her relationship with God has deepened. One caregiver stated that a consistent prayer life helped her to deal with her husband's injury. Another survivor stated that she became aware of how dependent she was on God's grace and forgiveness through the ordeal of the trial associated with her accident. Philippians 4:13 (NASB) became an anchor for another survivor of TBI, which says, "I can do all things through Him who strengthens me."

Scripture also speaks to creating purpose. Second Corinthians 5:17 (NASB) states, "Therefore if anyone is in Christ, he is a new creature; the old things passed away; behold new things have come." Faith in God appears to help survivors to create meaning out of their suffering and to share with others what they have learned. Ephesians 2:10 (NIV) reminds the believer, "For we are God's handiwork, created in Christ Jesus to do good works, which God prepared in advance for us to do." Brain injury does not eliminate God's plans. In fact, it just may be that God is using brain injury to encourage, equip, and educate others who have had a similar experience. Job, who experienced great losses of his family and fortune, said to God in Job 42:2 (NIV), "I know that you can do all things; no purpose of yours can be thwarted." And Psalm 138:8a (ESV) says that, "The Lord will fulfill his purpose for me; your steadfast love, O Lord, endures forever." Another promise that God will help someone fulfill his/her purpose is in Philippians 1:6 (NIV), which says, "I am sure of this, that he who began a good work in you will bring it to completion at the day of Jesus Christ." Psalm

57:2 (ESV) says, "I cry out to God Most High, to God who fulfills his purpose for me." The recognition that his/her injury may create purpose helps survivors to move beyond the mindset of limitations to the perspective of possibilities. The counselor has a rich opportunity to help survivors find their place in the world and live out their calling. It may be a different purpose than the survivor originally thought, but it will be exactly what is needed to provide hope, self-esteem, and purpose.

Conclusion

The experience of a brain injury in whatever form (acquired or traumatic) forces one to re-create one's self-concept and purpose in life. As Frankl (1968) suggested, adversity may strip away one's capability and dignity, but it cannot steal one's ability to choose. This chapter addressed the choice of creating a new self-concept after brain injury. The roles of returning to work, the community, and meaningful activity were explored as they relate to the development of purpose. Finally, both faith- and non-faith-based counseling techniques for individuals will guide them to creating their own life meaning stemming from their own moral code and set of values. Biblical promises were identified that support the idea that one's purpose in life is not abandoned after injury but rather enhanced.

References

Bandura, A. (1977). Self-efficacy: Toward a unifying theory of behavioral change. *Psychological Review, 84*, 191–215.

Cattelani, R., Tanzi, F., Lombardi, F., & Mazzucchi, A. (2002). Competitive re-employment after severe traumatic brain injury: Clinical, cognitive and behavioural predictive variables. *Brain Injury, 16*(1), 51–64.

Chen, L. (1997), Grief as a transcendent function and teacher of spiritual growth. *Pastoral Psychology, 46*(2), 79–84.

Cicerone, K. (1989). Psychotherapeutic interventions with traumatically brain-injured patients. *Rehabilitation Psychology, 34*(2), 105–114.

Donker-Cools, B., Schouten, M., Wind, H., & Frings-Dresen, M. (2018). Return to work following acquired brain injury: The views of patients and employers. *Disability and Rehabilitation, 40*(2), 185–191. https://doi.org/10.1080/09638288.2016.1250118

Douglas, J. (2013). Conceptualizing self and maintaining social connection following severe traumatic brain injury. *Brain Injury, 27*, 60–74.

Elbaum, J. (2007). Counseling individuals post acquired brain injury: Considerations and objectives. In J. Elbaum & D. Benson (Eds.), *Acquired brain injury: An integrative neuro-rehabilitation approach* (pp. 259–274). Springer.

Emmons, R., & McCullogh, M. (2003). Counting blessings versus burdens: Experimental studies of gratitude and subjective well-being in daily life. *Journal of Personality and Social Psychology, 84*(2), 377–389.

Fadyl, J., Theadom, A., Channon, A., & McPherson, K. (2019). Recovery and adaptation after traumatic brain injury in New Zealand: Longitudinal qualitative findings over the first two years. *Neuropsychological Rehabilitation, 29*(7), 1095–1112. https://doi.org/10.1080/09602011.2017.1364653

Frankl, V. (1968). *Man's search for meaning*. First Washington Square Press.

Godwin, E., & Kreutzer, J. (2013). Embracing a new path to emotional recovery: Adopting resilience theory in post-TBI psychotherapy. *Brain Injury, 27*(6), 637–639.

Hawthorne, G., Gruen, R., & Kaye, A. (2009). Traumatic brain injury and long-term quality of life: Findings from an Australian study. *Journal of Neurotrauma, 26*, 1623–1633.

Hoofien, D., Gilboa, A., Vakil, E., & Donovick, P. (2001). Traumatic brain injury (TBI) 10–20 years later: A comprehensive outcome study of psychiatric symptomology, cognitive abilities and psychosocial functioning. *Brain Injury, 15*(3), 189–209.

Iverson, G. (2012). A biopsychosocial conceptualization of poor outcome from mild traumatic brain injury. In J. Vasterling, R. Bryant, & T. Keane (Eds.), *PTSD and mild traumatic brain injury* (pp. 37–60). Guilford Press.

Johnstone, B., Yoon, D., Rupright, J., & Reid-Arndt, S. (2009). Relationships among spiritual beliefs, religious practices, congregational support and health for individuals with traumatic brain injury. *Brain Injury, 23*, 411–419.

Klonoff, P. (2010). *Psychotherapy after brain injury: Principles and techniques*. Guilford Press.

Knox, L., Douglas, J., & Bigby, C. (2017). "I've never been a yes person": Decision-making participation and self-conceptualization after severe traumatic brain injury. *Disability and Rehabilitation, 39*(22), 2250–2260. https://doi.org/10.1080/09638288.2016.1219925

Kreutzer, J., & Sander, A. (1997). Issues to brain injury evaluation and treatment. *Rehabilitation Psychology, 42*(3), 231–239.

Krych, D., & Schmidt, M. (2015). Beyond the evidence: What have we learned? Beyond the evidence: What do we believe? *Brain Injury Professional, 12*(1), 12–13.

Lennon, A., Bramham, J., Carroll, A., McElligott, J., Carton, S., Waldron, B., Fortune, D., Burke, T., Fitzhenry, M., & Benson, C. (2014). A qualitative exploration of how individuals reconstruct their sense of self following acquired brain injury in comparison with spinal cord injury. *Brain Injury, 28*(1), 27–37. https://doi.org/10.3109/02699052.2013.848378

Nyman, A., Kassberg, A., & Lund, M. (2021). Perceived occupational value in people with acquired brain injury. *Scandinavian Journal of Occupational Therapy, 28*(5), 391–398. https://doi.org/10.1080/11038128.2020.1791951

Olofsson, A., Lund, M., & Nyman, A. (2020). Everyday activities outside the home are a struggle: Narratives from two persons with acquired brain injury. *Scandinavian Journal of Occupational Therapy, 27*(3), 194–203. https://doi.org/10.1080/11038128.2018.1495762

Payne, L., Hawley, L., Ketchum, J., Philippus, A., Eagye, C., Morey, C., Gerber, D., Harrison-Felix, C., & Diener, E. (2018). Psychological well-being in individuals living in the community with traumatic brain injury. *Brain Injury, 32*(8), 980–985. https://doi.org/10.1080/02699052.2018.1468573

Ruff, R., & Chester, S. (2014). *Effective psychotherapy for individuals with brain injury*. Guilford Press.

Shigaki, C., Johnstone, B., & Schopp, L. (2009). Financial and vocational outcomes 2 years after traumatic brain injury. *Disability and Rehabilitation, 31*(6), 484–489.

Tsaousides, T., Warshowsky, A., Ashman, T., Cantor, J., Spielman, L., & Gordon, W. (2009). The relationship between employment-related self-efficacy and quality of life following traumatic brain injury. *Rehabilitation Psychology, 54*(3), 299–305.

Vickery, C., Gontkovsky, S., Wallace, J., & Caroselli, J. (2006). Group psychotherapy focusing on self-concept change following acquired brain injury: A pilot investigation. *Rehabilitation Psychology, 51*(1), 30–35.

Waldron-Perrine, B., Neils-Strunjas, J., Paul, D., Clark, A., Mudar, R., Maestas, K., Duff, M., & Bechtold, K. (2019). Integrating resilience-building into the neurorehabilitation process. *Brain Injury Professional, 16*(1), 28–31.

Winkler, D., Unsworth, C., & Sloan, S. (2006). Factors that lead to successful community integration following severe traumatic brain injury. *Journal of Head Trauma Rehabilitation, 21*, 8–21.

Winslade, W. (1998). *Confronting traumatic brain injury: Devastation, hope, and healing*. Yale University Press.

Index

Note: Page numbers in italics indicate figures.